# Sociological Perspectives on the New Genetics

# *Sociology of Health and Illness* Monograph Series

Edited by Jonathan Gabe
Department of Social and Political Social Science
Royal Holloway
University of London

**Current titles:**

*Medicine, Health and Risk*
Edited by Jonathan Gabe

*Health and the Sociology of Emotions*
Edited by Veronica James and Jonathan Gabe

*The Sociology of Medical Science and Technology*
Edited by Mary Ann Elston

*The Sociology of Health Inequalities*
Edited by Mel Bartley, David Blane and George Davey Smith

*Sociological Perspectives on the New Genetics*
Edited by Peter Conrad and Jonathan Gabe

**Forthcoming titles:**

*Rethinking the Sociology of Mental Health*
Edited by Joan Busfield

*Sociological Perspectives on Health Care Rationing*
Edited by Donald Light and David Hughes

# Sociological Perspectives on the New Genetics

Edited by Peter Conrad and Jonathan Gabe

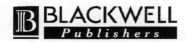

BLACKWELL
*Publishers*

Copyright © Blackwell Publishers Ltd/Editorial Board 1999

ISBN 0-631-21599-9

First published in 1999

Blackwell Publishers Ltd
108 Cowley Road, Oxford OX4 1JF, UK
and
350 Main Street
Malden, MA 02148, USA

*British Library Cataloguing in Publication Data*

A CIP catalogue record for this book is available from the British Library

*Library of Congress Cataloging-in-Publication Data*

applied for

Printed in Great Britain by MPG Books, Bodmin, Cornwall
This book is printed on acid-free paper.

# Acknowledgements

We should like to thank all those involved in the various stages of producing this monograph. We are grateful to the individual contributors for generally responding swiftly to deadlines, comments and queries. The anonymous referees who read each of the chapters, usually two or three times, have helped the contributors and ourselves enormously. We are especially indebted to Mary Ann Elston for support and advice. Anthea Holmes's copy-editing and Susan Gregory's administrative and proof-reading skills have also been invaluable.

# Contents

# Introduction: Sociological perspectives on the new genetics: an overview

*Peter Conrad and Jonathan Gabe*

We are at the dawn of a genetic age. The Human Genome Project, the largest biological research enterprise in history, promises to have our entire genetic structure mapped by 2001. Our media report new scientific claims of genes associated with diseases, conditions, behaviours or personality traits so regularly that it seems that we are being provided with a gene-of-the-week. Scientists have identified or claimed genes for cystic fibrosis, Huntington Disease, Fragile X syndrome, breast cancer, Alzheimer's disease, colon cancer, bipolar illness, obesity, homosexuality, alcoholism, 'novelty seeking', shyness, bed wetting; the list gets longer weekly. James Watson, co-discoverer of the double helix structure of DNA and founding father of the Human Genome Project has declared, 'We used to think our fate was in the stars. Now we know, in large part, it is in our genes' (cited in Horgan 1993).

The history of genetics is long and complex, encompassing numerous strands. In 1859 Gregor Mendel, an Austrian monk, discovered the rules of inheritance by doing carefully controlled breeding experiments with garden pea plants. In 1883 British scientist Frances Galton coined the term eugenics as 'the science of improvement of the human race germplasm through better breeding' (cited in Haller 1963: 3). For several decades eugenics thrived as both a form of 'science' and as a social movement. With the 'rediscovery' of Mendel's laws at the turn of the century, the eugenic movement adopted a scientific mantle and prospered in both the US and UK. Attempts at eugenic hygiene included identifying 'genetic defectives', and controlling their procreation or assimilation into society through marriage and immigration laws as well as sterilisation of 'undesirables'. In addition, eugenicists offered incentives for those deemed more generally fit (i.e. the upper classes) to increase their reproduction in order to improve the genetic stock. Prior to World War II, scientists and eugenicists proffered hereditarian theories of various diseases, conditions and behaviours. The eugenics movement flourished through the 30s, but eventually began to wane. Geneticists moved to separate themselves from the pseudo-science of eugenics, social scientists criticised the eugenicists' faulty underlying assumptions, and the Nazis' adoption of racist eugenic policies which led to the murder of millions, contributed to the demise of eugenic popularity (see Kevles 1985; Paul 1997). By the 1950s the term 'eugenics' had fallen into disrepute in the US and UK, and became a cautionary tale of the dangers of biased and bad science.

For much of the 20th century, scientific genetic research was limited to experiments on fruit flies and other laboratory experimental animals. There was little research on human genetics, and what there was was limited largely to twin and adoption studies. The emergence of the 'new genetics' can be marked by Watson and Crick's 1953 discovery of the double helix structure of DNA. This set the stage for the emergence of a new field, 'molecular biology', and the eventual development of research on genetic structure. By the 1980s molecular biology was a vast and vigorous field at the cutting edge of science. Genetic research received a huge infusion of funds and energy from the advent of the Human Genome Project, whose goal is to map the entire three billion base pairs of the human genetic structure. The purpose of the Genome Project is to find the chemical or genetic base for the 4000 or so genetic diseases that affect humans, as well as to identify genetic linkages with other diseases, with the hope of eventually creating new preventions and cures (Conrad 1997). With the introduction of new technologies, the genome project is progressing ahead of its original schedule. At this point, genetics is a rising paradigm in medicine and science. As the project proceeds, new claims about genetic associations and linkages with diseases, conditions and behaviours will be increasingly forthcoming over the next decade. Along with producing some remarkable discoveries, the new genetics engenders fresh concerns about legal and ethical issues (Kelves and Hood 1992; Kitcher 1996).

The mapping of the human genome has been the object of several provocative metaphors, including a search for the 'holy grail' (Gilbert 1992), investigating 'the essence of human life', and decoding 'the book of life'. Some critics have suggested that the gene is becoming a cultural icon in American society (Nelkin and Lindee 1995), invested with almost mystical powers. Others contend that the 'geneticisation' of human problems has expanded beyond scientific knowledge (Lippman 1992) and that a kind of 'genetic fatalism'—assuming that a genetic association is deterministic and a trait or behaviour is unchangeable—underlies much public discourse about genetics (Alper and Beckwith 1995). What is clear is that genetic research is relevant to an increasing number of diseases, conditions and behaviours, and that the genetic 'frame' is becoming common for explaining a wider range of human problems (Conrad 1997; Van Dijck 1998).

Scientists have already made brilliant discoveries of genes associated with diseases, yet the power of genetic knowledge can be overstated. Identifying the genes for cystic fibrosis and Huntington Disease are clearly major achievements, although as yet neither has generated new treatments for the disorders. Locating the BRCA1 and BRCA2 genes for breast cancer were remarkable breakthroughs, although they account for less than 10 per cent of all breast cancer. Discovered genes for bipolar illness, alcoholism, and novelty-seeking were widely heralded in the American and British media, only to be later disconfirmed when other scientists failed to replicate the results (Conrad 1997). Scientists will discover significant genetic associations with diseases in the next few years, some of which may result in preventions or treatments that may reduce human suffering. While the implications of finding genes for behaviour are less clear, there is little doubt that scientific reports of new genetic predispositions or causes of behaviours will be commonplace in the new millennium. Moreover, various types of genetic 'choice', from sex selection to personality traits to enhanced abilities, may become available through 'gene therapy', genetic reproductive technologies or human cloning. But at the dawn of the age of genetics, the genetic future is largely uncharted territory.

The new genetics revolution has ramifications far beyond the esoteric science of molecular biological laboratories. Technically 'gene' stands for a stretch of DNA that codes for protein. While genetics is fundamental for understanding human heredity, physiology and development, its social and cultural uses have expanded far beyond scientific knowledge. The rising genetic paradigm is influencing how we think about life, including disease and disability, human capacities and failings, social problems, kinship and the quality of life.

At the moment the public discourse about genetics outdistances validated scientific knowledge. Much of the public discourse around genetics assumes that scientists discover genes for a particular disease or behaviour; the complexity of genetic association and causation is glossed over when the media write about the 'gay gene' or the 'obesity gene'. It is as if there were an oversimplified Mendelian assumption, termed O-GOD (one gene, one disease), which involves a direct and virtual one-to-one relationship between genetics and behaviour (Conrad 1999). This clearly privileges genetic factors in the discourse, suggesting that genetics is the primary cause of a problem, when it may only be contributory. While it is likely that genetics plays a part in many human diseases and some behaviours, many of the early claims seem to exaggerate its importance.

## Sociology of genetics

We are also witnessing the dawn of the sociological study of the new genetics. While a few pioneers began work in the 1980s, the majority of sociological work on genetics has been published in the 1990s. Although sociological research on genetics is growing, the number of sociologists researching genetics is small compared, for example, with those who study problems like HIV/AIDS or stress and mental health. Here we touch briefly on the extant sociological work on genetics. Two caveats are in order: (1) the work noted here is representative rather than comprehensive of sociological interests;[1] and (2) given space limitations, in most cases we will only be able to identify the work rather than discuss it fully or critically.

One major focus has been to examine genetic counselling as a profession and the associated dilemmas of counsellor–client interaction. Bosk (1992)

presented an ethnographic account of genetic counselling at work, empha-
sising the perspective of the counsellors and focusing both on
professional–client and professional–colleague relations. His data are
grounded in the early days of the profession, when all the counsellors were
physicians. Today, in the US at least, most genetic counselling is done by
graduates or special genetic counselling Masters' Programs. Bosk highlights
some of the dilemmas of the genetic counselling position, especially the
desire to be value-neutral and non-directive. Several other sociologists have
studied genetic counselling work, most often from the perspective of clients
(Beeson 1997; Burke and Kolker 1993; Kolker and Burke 1994a, 1994b),
frequently focusing directly on the dilemmas of prenatal diagnosis (e.g.
Rothman 1986, 1996). Kenen has examined genetic counselling as a profession from its inception to its institutionalisation (1984, 1986, 1997). Wertz
(1992, 1994) has written a series of papers based on a 37-country survey of
geneticists and counsellors, examining and comparing their perspectives on
a range of bioethical issues.

Several sociologists have examined the public images and discourse
around the new genetics. Nelkin and Lindee (1995) investigated popular
images of genetics using an eclectic array of popular and professional
media as data—including film, television, news, ads, and books—to
analyse how depictions of genes are manifested in texts and images in popular culture. They show how groups appropriate the gene for their own
needs and argue that the gene has become something of a 'cultural icon'.
They contend that the increase in genetic explanations has given rise to a
'genetic essentialism', where the self or problem is reduced to a molecular
entity and located in genes. This is linked to the broader process of geneticisation (Lippman 1992), whereby an increasing range of human problems
is defined as genetic in origin. Conrad (Conrad and Weinberg 1996,
Conrad 1997) has examined specifically how genetics and behaviour are
depicted in the news; he shows how the news media often misrepresent scientific reality by adopting a frame of 'genetic optimism' and not reporting
ensuing disconfirmations, leading to a privileging of genetics in public discourse. Rothman's (1998) recent popular account focuses on the ways in
which genetics has shaped the lens through which we see the world. Duster
(1990) has suggested that we are increasingly seeing problems through a
'prism of heredity'.

Related to the public discourse about genetics are analyses that explore
lay and professional perspectives on genetics and heredity. Some significant
work has been done on this topic by Kerr et al. (1997, 1998). Based on interviews and focus groups, Kerr and her colleagues found that the lay public
was knowledgeable about genetics but had a different (e.g. experientially-
based) knowledge from professionals. Richards (1996), on the other hand,
contends that the public understanding of Mendelian genetics is very limited, and suggests that Mendelian genetics conflicts with lay knowledge of
inheritance which is grounded in everyday understandings of kinship. Other

analysts have investigated the impact of differential lay understanding on 'risk' (Parsons and Atkinson, 1992 1993; Hallowell and Richards 1997) and how these differential understandings might affect behaviour and choice (Davison 1996). Both lay and professional understandings about genetics are based on experience and social location. Yet professionals see their perspectives as objective, and often dismiss lay perspectives, at the same time deflecting ultimate responsibility for the use of genetic knowledge (Kerr et al. 1997). The lay–professional disjunction of understanding has important implications for medical and policy decisions about genetics; interestingly, however, this issue has received considerable sociological attention in the UK and much less elsewhere.

The spectre for eugenics casts a shadow over the new genetics. The eugenic misuses and abuses of earlier this century, including immigration restriction, institutionalisation, sterilisation and the Nazi genocide, have been recounted by historians (e.g. Kevles 1985; Rafter 1992; Paul 1997). While the new genetics is more medical, involves committed individual choice, and has not led to overtly discriminatory state policies, the pall of eugenic history is reflected in anxieties about genetics. Duster (1990) focuses on the social implications of screening for inherited genetic disorders, especially those that are differentially distributed by race and ethnicity. Although Duster does not see the imminent rise of eugenics in its earlier misdirected and malevolent forms, he suggests that we may have a 'back-door to eugenics' in the name of health through screens, treatments and therapies. While most genetic professionals distance themselves from the abuses and 'bad science' of the old eugenics (Kerr et al. 1998), several sociologists raise concerns about potential eugenic outcomes due to prenatal screening for devalued traits (e.g. disabilities) (Shakespeare 1995) or the enhancement of humans through embryo genetic manipulation (Steinberg 1997). Individual choice and disincentives (e.g. by insurance coverage) may engender eugenics by outcome rather than by policy intent. This may be subtler but could be equally pernicious. Although short of actual eugenics, associating race or ethnicity with certain genes could lead to forms of genetic discrimination (e.g. Dyson 1998).

Sociologists have researched other areas of genetics, including the social construction of genetic knowledge (Atkinson et al. 1997; Conrad 1999), the emergence and implications of genetic testing (Nelkin 1997; Draper 1994), the social control potential of genetic information (Nelkin and Tancredi 1989) and the commercialisation of genetic bio-technology (Martin 1995). Feminist sociologists studying reproductive technology have contributed significantly to our understanding of genetics in this context (e.g. Rothman 1998; Steinberg 1997), especially in terms of the implications of prenatal diagnosis and the potentials of reproductive technology (e.g. Rothman 1986; Kolker and Burke 1993).[2]

We have probably imposed more order on sociological work about the new genetics than most of the authors would claim, but the attempt here was to display some of the major issues that have come under sociological investigation. The sociological study of genetics is still in its infancy; it will undoubtedly continue to grow as impacts of the new genetics become more clear. One of the challenges will be to find or create appropriate sociological frameworks for understanding genetics and its implications. While it seems clear that sociological perspectives can enlighten our understanding of genetics and its place in society, it is not always apparent how the study of genetics can contribute to sociology. This must be one of our intellectual challenges as we enter the new millennium.

## Overview of this issue

This is the first volume to draw together a range of sociological perspectives on the new genetics. The chapters included here are loosely organised around three themes, which intersect and advance some of the foci we have identified above in the extant sociological work on genetics. The chapters under our first theme examine how genetic knowledge is produced and structured, which includes professional perspectives and public images. Our second theme expands previous work on genetic counselling and lay perspectives, focusing on social meanings of genetics. The final theme elaborates on a continuing sociological interest, the implications of the new genetics for society.

### Theme 1: The structure and production of genetic knowledge

Genetic knowledge does not emerge solely by applying a set of scientific procedures to problems of the body, the structure of DNA, or identifying patterns of inheritance. Cultural assumptions shape what kinds of questions scientists ask, where they look for answers and how they interpret their data. Why, for example, have scientists searched for the genetic basis of homosexuality rather than heterosexuality, for alcoholism but not caffeine addiction, or for IQ but not musical ability? What genetic knowledge is sought, who seeks it, whose claims are honoured, and how genetic data are interpreted reflect cultural assumptions and social values. How do problems become geneticised and with what consequences? Sociologists, especially those working within a social constructionist framework, are well equipped to ask such questions.

In 'Genes as drugs: the social shaping of gene therapy and the reconstruction of genetic disease', Paul Martin uses a sociology of technology framework to examine the development of gene therapy in the United States. He shows how the perception of what constitutes genetic disease changed during the introduction of gene therapy. Scientists broadened their focus from the relatively rare inherited disorders that resulted from genetic defects to include more common diseases, like heart disease and cancer, which could be deemed to have a genetic component. Some also included behavioural disorders such as alcoholism and mental illness. This expanded the notion of the 'genetic body' and created a wider potential for the introduction of gene therapy. The interaction among scientists, clinicians and the pharmaceutical industry reshaped the notion of what constitutes a genetic problem and created new possibilities for genetic medical treatment.

What is a genetic problem is not always self-evident. Elizabeth Ettorre interviewed experts in four European countries to ascertain their perceptions of reproductive genetics. In her chapter, 'Experts as "storytellers" in reproductive genetics: exploring key issues', she analyses how experts construct families and genetic knowledge in the 'stories' they create about prenatal diagnosis. She argues that these stories produce 'genetic ideologies' about what types of families are in need of prenatal genetic screening. These ideologies include who are 'normal patients', i.e. families with a genetic problem. According to Ettorre, many experts believe that it is empowering for families to know their genetic make-up as it enables clearer reproductive choices. This may not always be the case, since lay understandings inevitably encompass other contextual issues (see articles discussed under Theme 2). In the second part of the chapter, Ettorre outlines some strategies experts use to substantiate their claims about the salience of genetic knowledge and their expertise.

The media are central to the public understanding of genetics. But the media do not simply report scientific findings; they are selective in their coverage, and construct genetics for public consumption. In 'The human drama of genetics: "hard" and "soft" media representations of inherited breast cancer', Lesley Henderson and Jenny Kitzinger examine news and popular coverage of 'breast cancer genes' (BRCA1 and BRCA2). They compare 'hard' news accounts in newspapers with 'soft' human interest stories in women's magazines and television fiction. Although less than 10 per cent of the disease occurrence can be attributed to breast cancer genes, the genetic/inherited risk of breast cancer has received a good deal of media attention. The dilemmas of women in 'high risk families' are common fare for popular press and television. These stories privilege genetics and amplify the idea that breast cancer is a genetic disease far beyond its epidemiological reality. The authors conclude that media values rather than scientific findings promote certain types of presentations of genetic information; with the increase of 'soft' media approaches, these may become the public's main source of information.

*Theme 2: The social meanings of genetics*
Genetics is a scientific discipline for understanding inheritance in living things. But the meanings of genetics, and the understanding people have about genetics, are not given in the biological genetic structure or our knowledge about the operation of genes. Social meanings involve interpretation and thus can vary by culture, group or situation. Thus genetic understandings can vary greatly, depending where one looks.

Alan Stockdale, in 'Waiting for the cure: mapping the social relations of human gene therapy research', shows a wide gulf between scientific and lay views of genetic therapy. Investigating the case of cystic fibrosis (CF), he argues that researchers and their supporters have over-sold the current efficacy of gene therapy (or gene transfer) and have raised public expectations of immediate success. In part this is based on a disjunction between scientists' and patients' experience. But it is not only scientists; Stockdale specifically implicates the Cystic Fibrosis Foundation for the strategies it uses in raising funds. The CFF's fund-raising strategy centres on the idea that scientists are near a 'cure' for this 'child-killer'. But the gene therapy cure is not at hand, and CF is no longer the child-killer it was two decades ago; individuals with CF now frequently live into their 30s (and discovery of the CF gene has had no effect on this). While gene therapy may offer treatments in the future, it has little meaning for those currently affected by the disease.

When a disease is defined as genetic it moves from an individual to a family disease. In recent years it has become clear that some forms of breast and ovarian cancer are hereditary. In 'Doing the right thing: genetic risk and responsibility', Nina Hallowell examines the perceptions and behaviours around risk among women at a genetic counselling clinic for hereditary breast and ovarian cancer. She found that the women generally perceived themselves at risk of cancer. Their behaviour, however, was not only based on their perceptions of risk but was profoundly influenced by their sense of obligation to other family members (dead, alive and unborn). Many of these women espoused an ethic of genetic responsibility to others which meant they were prepared to compromise their own needs of 'not knowing' for the sake of others. Hallowell suggests that genetic risk becomes a moral issue that can constrain rather than expand women's options and choices. Given the plethora of evidence that women often put others' needs above their own, it would be interesting to see if the same type of genetic responsibility was evident in a cohort of men at a colon cancer clinic. To what extent does gender affect the perceptions of and responses to genetic risk?

The O-GOD (one gene, one disease) model of disease is appropriate only in selected single gene disorders. Huntington Disease (HD) is one of these; if an individual carries the gene, and lives long enough, s/he will develop the disease. For over a decade there has been a predictive test for HD. In '"There's this thing in our family": predictive testing and the social construction of risk for Huntington Disease', Sue M. Cox and William H. McKellin explore the meaning and significance of hereditary risk for HD in everyday life. They show how the perception of risk emerges in family interaction, creating a jointly constructed meaning of 'this thing' in the family. This lay construction of risk is not necessarily informed by a Mendelian theory of inheritance but is based on issues like social or geographic proximity. These meanings shape the experience and impact of predictive testing. This article provides an excellent example of the processes and consequences of the interaction of social and biological knowledge in creating a perception of hereditary risk.

*Theme 3: The social impact and implications of genetics*

The greatest concerns about the new genetics inhere in the potential social impacts and implications. Advocates and critics alike have raised concerns about the implications of genetics, albeit with different emphases. Among the more important implications so far identified, we include: the privacy of genetic information, the potential of genetic stigmatisation and discrimination, geneticisation and the privileging of genetic explanations, the extent and role of genetic screening, genetic interventions in reproduction (especially in terms of in vitro fertilisation, gene therapy, enhancements and the spectre of cloning), and the perils of new forms of eugenics. Which social implications are most significant varies by who is examining what from which perspective.

While there is by now a clear consensus that the new genetics has social implications, there is less agreement on what those implications might be. In 'Defining the "social": towards an understanding of scientific and medical discourses on the social aspects of the new genetics', Sarah Cunningham-Burley and Anne Kerr examine how the social aspects of genetics are depicted in the scientific and clinical literature. They argue that through their writings scientists are influential parties who focus on the beneficial social implications of genetics, at the same time marginalising the more critical commentaries. The scientists' writings provide a form of rhetorical boundary marking between science and society, protecting their cognitive authority from challenging discourses. This suggests that the role of sociologists and bioethicists in creating independent and critical analysis of the social implications cannot be overstated.

The perceptions of the potential impact of the new genetics can vary for different stake-holders in the genetic world. Tom Shakespeare, in '"Losing the Plot"? Medical and activist discourses of contemporary genetics and disability', contrasts claims in the medical genetic discourse with the critique by disability activists. While the medical discourse is optimistic about genetics and distances itself from eugenic aims, disability activists worry that genetic interventions will lead inevitably to a new form of eugenics. Shakespeare finds that both discourses tend to overstate the potential of genetics to impact the lives of people with disabilities. Yet the issues of public health goals and perspectives of disability activists may continue to clash, with the activists claiming that genetic intervention of disabilities negates the value of disabled people and medical advocates saying they want to prevent disabilities, not people. But genetic interventions, such as selective abortion or gene therapy, may lead to a eugenics by outcome if not by intent.

Some impacts of genetics have wider social implications. Numerous scientists and supporters of genetics suggest that before long all of us will carry Genome cards encoded with DNA chips that will allow rapid medical access to our genetic endowment. While these are not yet viable, other forms of genetic identification are. In 'Genetic identification and surveillance creep', Dorothy Nelkin and Lori Andrews discuss some of the ramifications of DNA testing. We each have a unique genomic structure. DNA testing is non-intrusive and currently widely available; it requires only a small piece of hair, saliva, blood or semen. It has been used for criminal DNA fingerprinting, paternity determinationation and identifying missing children, biological relatives, and dead bodies. The military and government want to create large DNA databases for a variety of purposes. While there are some legitimate uses for DNA testing, Nelkin and Andrews view the expansion of mandatory genetic testing with concern, seeing it as broadening the range of public surveillance. Who will have access to the data, how will it be used, and what is the impact on privacy? From a sociological perspective, we need to ask how genetic testing can become a form of social control, with what consequences for society and the individual. This provides an important reminder that issues around genetics are not limited to those with genetic disorders or identified genetic susceptibilities, but rather the new genetics is likely to affect all of us.

## Acknowledgment

Thanks to Emily Kolker for her comments on an earlier draft of this introduction.

## Notes

1   We limit our discussion to sociologists or articles published in sociological journals; anthropologists including Rayna Rapp, Deborah Heath, Karen-Sue Taussig, and Margaret Lock, among others, have also written relavent pieces on the new genetics.
2   We focus primarily on sociological studies of the new genetics. However, sociologists have also written important critical analyses of the claims about 'race, genes and IQ' and of sociobiology, neither of which we have the space to include here.

## References

Alper, J.S. and Beckwith, J. (1993) Genetic fatalism and social policy: the implications of behavior genetics research, *Yale Journal of Biology and Medicine*, 66, 511–24.
Atkinson, P., Butcher, C. and Parsons, E. (1997) The rhetoric of prediction and chance in the research to clone a disease gene. In Elston, M.A. (ed) *The Sociology of Medical Science and Technology*. Oxford: Blackwell.
Beeson, D. (1997) Nuance, complexity and context: qualitative methods in genetic counselling research, *Women and Health*, 23, 21–43.

Bosk, C.K. (1992) All God's Mistakes: Genetic Counseling in a Pediatric Hospital. Chicago: University of Chicago Press.

Burke, B.M. and Kolker, A. (1993) Clients undergoing chorionic villus sampling versus amniocentesis: contrasting attitudes toward pregnancy, *Health Care for Women International*, 13, 103–200.

Conrad, P. (1997) Public eyes and private genes: historical frames, news constructions and social problems, *Social Problems*, 44, 139–54.

Conrad, P. (1999) A mirage of genes, *Sociology of Health and Illness*, 21, 2, 228–39.

Conrad, P. and Weinberg, D. (1996) Has the gene for alcoholism been discovered three times since 1980? a news media analysis, *Perspectives on Social Problems*, 8, 3–24.

Davison, C. (1996) Predicting genetics: the cultural implications of supplying probable futures. In Marteau, T. and Richard, M.P.M. (eds) *The Troubled Helix: Social and Psychological Implications of the New Human Genetics*. Cambridge: Cambridge University Press.

Draper, E. (1994) *Risky Business*. Berkeley: University of California Press.

Duster, T. (1990) *Backdoor to Eugenics*. New York: Routledge.

Dyson, S. (1998) 'Race', ethnicity and haemoglobin disorders, *Social Science and Medicine*, 47, 121–31.

Gilbert, W. (1992) A vision of the holy grail. In Kelves, D. and Hood, L. (eds) The Code of Codes. Cambridge: Harvard University Press

Haller, M.H. (1963) *Eugenics: Hereditarian Attitudes in American Thought*. New Brunswick, NJ: Rutgers University Press.

Hallowell, N. and Richard, M.P.M. (1997) Understanding life's lottery: an evaluation of studies of genetic risk awareness, *Journal of Health Psychology*, 2, 31–43.

Horgan, J. (1993) Eugenics revisited, *Scientific American*, 269, June, 122–31.

Kenen, R. (1984) Genetic counseling: the development of a new interdisciplinary field, *Social Science and Medicine*, 18, 541–59.

Kenen, R. (1986) Growing pains of a new health care field: genetic counseling in Australia and the United States, *Australian Journal of Social Issues*, 21, 172–82.

Kenen, R. (1997) Opportunities and impediments for a consolidating and expanding profession: genetic counseling in the United States, *Social Science and Medicine*, 45: 1377–86.

Kerr, A., Cunningham-Burley, S. and Amos, A. (1997) The new genetics: professionals' discursive boundaries, *The Sociological Review*, 35, 279–303.

Kerr, A., Cunningham-Burley, S. and Amos, A. (1998) The new genetics and health: mobilizing lay expertise, *Public Understanding of Science*, 7, 41–60.

Kevles, D.H. (1985) *In the Name of Eugenics: Genetics and the Uses of Human Heredity*. Berkeley: University of California Press.

Kevles, D. and Hood, L. (1991) Out of eugenics: the historical politics of the human genome. In Hood, L. and Kevles, D. (eds) *The Code of Codes*. Cambridge: Harvard University Press.

Kitcher, P. (1992) T*he Lives to Come: the Genetic Revolution and Human Possibilities*. New York: Simon and Schuster.

Kolker, A. and Burke, M.B. (1993) Sex preference and sex selection: attitudes of prenatal diagnosis clients, *Research in the Sociology of Health Care*, 10, 213–32.

Kolker, A. and Burke, M.B. (1994a) Prenatal Testing: a Sociological Perspective. Westport: Bergin and Garvey.

Kolker, A. and Burke, M.B. (1994b) Directiveness in prenatal genetic counseling, *Women and Health*, 22, 31–53.

Lippman, A. (1992) Led (astray) by genetic maps: the cartography of the human genome and health care, *Social Science and Medicine*, 35, 1469–76.

Martin, P. (1995) The American gene therapy industry and the social shaping of a new technology, *The Genetic Engineer and Biotechnologist*, 15, 155–67.

Nelkin, D. (1997) The social dynamics of genetic testing: the case of Fragile-X, *Medical Anthropology Quarterly*, 10, 537–50.

Nelkin, D. and Lindee, M.S. (1995) *The DNA Mystique: the Gene as a Cultural Icon*. New York: W.H. Freeman.

Nelkin, D. and Tancredi, L. (1989) *Dangerous Diagnostics: the Social Power of Biological Information*. New York: Basic Books.

Parsons, E. and Atkinson, P. (1992) Lay constructions of genetic risk, *Sociology of Health and Illness*, 14, 437–55.

Parsons, E. and Atkinson, P. (1993) Genetic risk and reproduction, *The Sociological Review*, 41, 679–706.

Paul, D. (1997), *Controlling Human Heredity*. New Jersey: Humanities Press.

Rafter, N. (1992) Claims-making and socio-cultural context in the first US eugenics campaign, *Social Problems*, 39, 17–34.

Richards, M.P.M. (1993) The new genetics—issues for social scientists, *Sociology of Health and Illness*, 567–86.

Richards, M.P.M. (1996) Lay and professional knowledge of genetics and inheritance, Public Understanding of Science, 5, 217–30.

Rothman, B.K. (1986) *Tentative Pregnancy: Prenatal Diagnosis and the Future of Motherhood*. New York: Norton.

Rothman, B.K. (1996) Of maps and imagination: sociology confronts the genome, *Social Problems*, 42, 1–10.

Rothman, B.K. (1998) *Genetic Maps and Human Imaginations: the Limits of Science in Understanding Who We Are*. New York: Norton.

Shakespeare, T. (1995) Back to the future? New genetics and disabled people, *Social Policy*, 46, 22–35.

Steinberg, D. L. (1997) *Bodies in Glass: Genetics, Eugenics, Embryo Ethics*. Manchester: Manchester University Press.

Van Dijck, J. (1998) *Imagination: Popular Images of Genetics*. New York: New York University Press.

Wertz, D. (1992) Ethical and legal implications of the new genetics: issues for discussion, *Social Science and Medicine*, 35, 495–505.

Wertz, D. (1994) Provider gender and moral reasoning: the politics of an 'ethics of care', *Journal of Genetic Counselling*, 3, 95–112.

# I: Structure and Production of Genetic Knowledge

# 1. Genes as drugs: the social shaping of gene therapy and the reconstruction of genetic disease

*Paul A. Martin*

## Introduction

The idea that diseases and bodies are socially and historically constructed is well established within both medical sociology and the history of medicine, and has inspired a great deal of research (Wright and Treacher 1982, Rosenberg and Golden 1997). Many different approaches have been used to examine the processes by which new medical knowledge is created, including studies of medical education, biomedical research and clinical practice. However, with some notable exceptions (Peitzman 1997, Lawrence 1997, Wailoo 1997), relatively little attention has been paid to the relationship between the development of new technologies, the formation of new medical knowledge and the way in which new disease concepts have arisen.

This omission is of particular concern in the area of modern genetics where the introduction of powerful new technologies is closely linked to the construction of new accounts about the origins of disease. In particular, the emergence of new forms of genetic determinism questions established social and environmental explanations of why people become ill and challenge existing views about the responsibility of both the individual and society. The rise of the new genetics also raises important questions within medical sociology about the role of technology and the nature of technical change within medicine, a topic that has been largely neglected until recently (Elston 1997). Studies within science and technology studies (STS) have, in contrast, started to examine some of these issues. In particular, a number of authors have investigated the ways in which new technologies and new medical knowledge are co-constructed (Saetnan 1991, Blume 1992, Clarke and Montini 1993, Koch and Stemerding 1994, Prout 1996, Oudshoorn 1994, Berg 1997).

One of the main consequences of the introduction of new genetic technologies has been a change within medicine in the type of explanations given about the cause of many diseases. Recent research in the history and sociology of medicine has started to analyse these new accounts and the way in which new biomedical knowledge is constructing a 'genetic body' (Koch 1993, Turney and Balmer 1998). In this discourse a number of relatively rare inherited conditions are the result of genetic defects, while other more common pathologies, such as heart disease, are seen to have a significant genetic component. In addition, claims are also being made about the genetic basis of behaviour 'disorders' such as depression, schizophrenia, and alcoholism. Within this conceptual framework, environmental and social factors may play a role in the onset of disease, but it is ultimately the genetic dowry we each inherit which determines our health status. However, this notion of how genes cause disease is historically constructed and is in no sense fixed or unchanging. This chapter will draw on work within the sociology of technology to analyse how the perception of what constitutes a genetic disease has changed during the introduction of a new medical technology, gene therapy, into experimental clinical practice. Gene therapy involves the transfer of genes into cells for the treatment of disease. By the end of 1996 the technology was being tested experimentally in over 2,000 patients in more than 160 human clinical trials in the USA alone and was being commercially developed by over 50 American firms (Martin and Thomas 1996). However, it must be stressed that even by 1999 no gene therapy had been proven to work in humans and no product was expected to get regulatory approval for routine clinical use before 2002.

It will be argued that in the field of gene therapy there has been a shift from an account of disease based on 'classical' genetics and the inheritance of deleterious genes, to one which explains many common acquired pathologies in terms of errors in the way gene are regulated. At the same time, however, this shift in the meaning of genetic disease has both depended on, and enabled, a fundamental change in the definition, applications and design of gene therapy technology itself. Over the course of 30 years it has been reshaped from being a largely surgical procedure for the treatment of rare inherited disorders to its introduction as a novel form of drug therapy for common acquired conditions.

It will also be shown that the changes in both the definition of genetic disease and the constitution of gene therapy were not just the result of new medical knowledge and discourses, or the introduction of novel forms of clinical work. They also rested on the creation of new socio-technical relations, new organisations and new artefacts, aligned into stable networks. Central to this process have been attempts by scientists to commercially exploit the technology through the creation of dedicated gene therapy firms. This chapter will therefore examine the historical development of gene therapy paying particular attention to the way it has been designed, applied in experimental clinical practice, and commercially developed by industry. By presenting an account based on the analysis of these socio-technical networks it is hoped that the chapter will demonstrate the utility of taking established concepts from STS and applying them to the traditional concerns of medical sociology.

# New knowledge, new technologies and the construction of socio-technical networks

In the last 15 years a new sociology of technology has started to be articulated, based on a critique of technological determinism (MacKenzie and Wajcman 1985, Bijker *et al.* 1987). Instead of innovation and technological change being driven by an innate technical logic, the development of new technologies is seen as a fundamentally social process open to sociological analysis.

A number of different theoretical perspectives have been used to examine the creation of new technologies, including actor-network theory (ANT) (Callon 1987), the social construction of technology (SCOT) (Bijker 1995) and the analysis of large technical systems (Hughes 1987). Although each takes a distinct approach they share several common features, notably the idea that the development of a new technology involves a range of heterogeneous social, technical, economic and political processes. In addition, it is argued that new knowledge is co-produced at the same time as new technologies and new socio-technical relations, through a process of mutual shaping.

This chapter will draw on the following concepts within this new sociology of technology:

*The construction of socio-technical networks*
In order to be successfully introduced into routine use new technologies require the alignment of a range of heterogeneous human and non-human actors into stable socio-technical networks (Callon 1987). To achieve this, network builders, or 'heterogeneous engineers', might be involved in, for example, the creation of new social practices, new companies and new forms of state regulation, which emerge together during innovation. Network formation therefore requires the enrolment of various actors, the formation of alliances and the mobilising of different social, technical, and economic resources.

*The creation of visions and the enrolment of support*
An important process in the formation of networks is the creation of particular 'visions' or expectations for how the technology might be used in practice and sold as a commodity (van Lente 1993). Visions act as both a means of enrolling support and resources into the emerging socio-technical network and as a guide to the physical design of artefacts. They may also form part of a new set of cognitive structures that both enable and shape the development of the technology (Bijker 1995). During the early stages in the introduction of a radically new technology a number of competing visions for how it might be used may co-exist (Pinch and Bijker 1984). These are often associated with the formation of different networks and the emergence of alternative designs or technological options.

*The social shaping of technology*
As an integral part of the creation of stable socio-technical networks the emerging technology is socially shaped to reflect the activities and interests of the groups involved in the innovation process. This is mediated through the design, testing, selection and redesign of the various technological options and may result in the physical form of the technology changing dramatically over time. For example, as new groups of actors join the emerging network, they may favour particular options over others and shape the future direction of research and design (Bijker 1995). Through an examination of the competing technological options, the changing designs and applications, and the role of the various groups involved, it thus becomes possible to analyse the physical development of a new technology in sociological terms.

These theoretical tools will be used to analyse the development of gene therapy in the United States (US) between the late 1950s and 1996. The US was chosen because almost all the work in this field took place in America before 1990 and the research draws on both historical documents and interviews with scientists, clinicians and the managers of gene therapy companies (Martin 1998). I shall start with a brief history of the early development of gene therapy and the work leading to the initial clinical trial of the technology in 1989. Case studies of different strategies for the subsequent introduction of gene therapy into experimental clinical practice will then be used to examine changes in both the concept of genetic disease and the design of the technology. Finally, I shall reflect on the socio-technical processes that have been at work, the way in which the idea of a genetic disease has been reconstituted and the manner in which gene therapy technology has been socially shaped during this period.

## The early development of gene therapy: from eugenics to therapeutics

*The construction of different technological options*
The idea of genetic therapy has its roots in pre-World War II futurism and eugenics. The first suggestions for the genetic alteration of people for both social and medical reasons can be found in the writings of scientists such as Haldane and Muller, and the science fiction of Stapledon (Haldane 1923, Muller 1935, Stapledon 1930). Early advocates of the technology drew on Jacques Loeb's concept of 'biological engineering' as a means of modifying man and combating the degeneration of the race (Pauly 1987). These ideas were also articulated in the policies and programmes of the Rockefeller Foundation, whose funding was fundamental in shaping the development of the new science of molecular biology during the 1930s and 40s (Kay 1993).

In many ways, biological engineering was implicit in the central project of molecular biology from its beginning, but it only found clear scientific expression with the advent of early gene transfer techniques after the War. The first programmatic proposal for genetic therapy was made in Edward Tatum's 1958 Nobel Prize acceptance speech in which he anticipated molecular biology enabling 'the improvement of all living organisms by processes which we might call biological engineering' (Tatum 1958: 75).

The idea of biological engineering was subsequently articulated by a number of the early scientific leaders of molecular biology, many of whom had worked on gene transfer in the 1940s and 50s (Hotchkiss 1965, Szybalski 1992). However, two competing 'visions' of how genetic therapy might be developed emerged during these first discussions of the subject during the 1960s. The first took its inspiration from eugenics and was centred on the idea of modifying future generations to make social and intellectual 'improvements' and cure genetic diseases. This vision was advocated by Hermann Muller and other supporters of what Kevles has called reform eugenics (Muller 1965). The second vision was purely medical and was only concerned with genetically altering affected patients and not their offspring (Tatum 1966). It was mainly proposed by a younger generation of clinically trained investigators who largely rejected the eugenics of the 1930s.[1]

Both these visions found expression in scientific research programmes aimed at inserting foreign genes into mammalian cells and drew on the recently developed techniques of recombinant DNA and funding from the National Institutes of Health (NIH). The realisation of the neo-eugenic vision depended on being able to transfer genes into sperm or eggs, the so-called germ cells, so that changes might be inherited by future generations. Several investigators attempted to develop techniques to alter germ cells during the late 1960s and early 70s, culminating in 1982 in the creation of the world's first 'transgenic' mouse which contained a growth hormone gene from the rat (Palmiter et al. 1982). In contrast, attempts to realise the medical vision rested on inserting genes into cells other than the sperm and eggs (the somatic tissues). In particular, research focused on the treatment of blood disorders such as thalassemia, where cells might be removed, genetically modified and returned to the patient using conventional blood transfusion. The alteration of cells outside the body became known as *ex vivo* therapy. This was in contrast to the direct injection of genes into the patient, so called *in vivo* therapy. Despite their different aims the neo-eugenic vision and the medical alternative were constructed around the central concept of classical genetics in which the inheritance of deleterious genes cause particular diseases.[2] Both options continued to be actively investigated by a small number of scientists until the early 1980s when a major new debate about the ethics of gene therapy started to fundamentally influence the direction of research.

*Opposition, ethics and the development of 'classical gene therapy'*
During the 1960s, scientific progress in molecular biology and reproductive technology prompted discussion in the media of a forthcoming 'biological revolution' (Turney 1998). At the time many of these new developments

were couched in positive futuristic terms, but by the 70s concern grew about the social and ethical consequences of 'playing god'. These included fears of creating a super race using genetic engineering and several prominent molecular biologists voiced their misgivings about the direction of research (Luria 1969). This unease coincided with a growing sense of environmental crisis, concern about the abuse of science and the anti-Vietnam War movement, and led to the formation of groups such as the Committee for Responsible Genetics. Public fears about genetic engineering were crystallised in 1980 when Martin Cline, a prominent American clinician, attempted the world's first human experiment using recombinant DNA techniques: an event which prompted the first organised opposition to the development of gene therapy (Cook-Deegan 1990).

Cline made international headlines for not only trying to cure thalassemia by genetically modifying the bone marrow of two patients, but also because he deliberately proceeded after being refused prior ethical approval for the research. The storm of protest that followed his experiment culminated in an inquiry into the ethics of gene therapy by the recently created President's Commission for the Study of Ethical Problems in Medicine, and Biomedical and Behavioral Research (the President's Commission) (Cook-Deegan 1990). The Commission findings were published in 1982 in the landmark report *Splicing Life*, coinciding with increasing political pressure for an outright ban on research into gene therapy from religious groups, environmental activists and a number of prominent scientists.

The Commission's report was important in making a distinction between the neo-eugenic idea of altering future generations, which it called germ line therapy, and the medical use of gene transfer directed solely at treating the non-reproductive cells of an individual patient, which it labelled somatic gene therapy. The Commission believed that germ line therapy was unethical and should not be allowed, but it felt it was acceptable to proceed with the development of somatic therapy for life threatening genetic diseases (President's Commission for the Study of Ethical Problems in Medicine and Biomedical and Behavioral Research 1982). This distinction subsequently played a key role in helping legitimise somatic therapy as little more than a conventional medical intervention and has shaped all subsequent debates about the ethics of gene therapy (Capron 1990). Furthermore, it also distanced the technology from eugenics and the idea of human genetic engineering and strengthened the association with therapy.

*Splicing Life*, and a subsequent study by the Congressional Office of Science and Technology, were then deliberately used by the advocates of gene therapy to enrol support amongst bioethicists, theologians and scientists around the idea of somatic therapy (Cook-Deegan 1990). In particular, politicians and government policy makers played a key role in the process of winning consent. As part of this process a de facto moratorium was placed on clinical research into gene therapy and in 1984 the National Institutes of Health Recombinant Advisory Committee ('the RAC') was given responsibility for establishing a regulatory framework for clinical research in this area which would attract broad public support.

The RAC was composed of a majority of scientists as well as clinicians, lawyers, policy makers and lay members, and as such brought together the key groups whose support had to be enrolled. It subsequently acted as the locus of an attempt by the scientific advocates of gene therapy to build a national consensus about what sort of research would be socially acceptable. This was not an easy process and it was only in 1986 that the Committee finalised its guidelines. Furthermore, the RAC's criteria for an experiment were demanding, and a trial would only be approved for ex vivo somatic therapy targeting a life threatening genetic disease for which there was no alternative cure (National Institutes of Health 1985).

Following *Splicing Life* all serious work on germ line therapy ceased and the field's sole attention rested on developing ways of transferring genes into blood stem cells, the immortal precursors of the entire blood and immune system. If this could be achieved it would then be possible to provide a permanent cure for a number of rare enzyme deficiencies and genetic disorders. This approach to gene therapy drew heavily on classical genetics and the concept of genetic diseases caused by single gene defects and simply aimed to replace or correct the gene that caused the condition. For this reason it became known as 'classical' gene therapy and dominated the field until 1984, with the prime disease target continuing to be thalassemia (Anderson 1984). However, around this time it became apparent that the efficient transfer of the globin gene, which caused the disease, was still a long way from being technically feasible. This was a major setback to the field and brought all plans for immediate clinical development to a halt (Martin 1998).

These technical difficulties severely limited the possibility of progress. During the mid-1980s gene therapy was still highly controversial, pursued by fewer than 10 laboratories in the USA. Furthermore, research was focused on a small number of very rare genetic diseases and commanded little interest amongst clinicians more generally. Despite this, the sanctioning of somatic therapy as ethical, the enrolment of support from theologians, bioethicists and politicians, and the formation of a socially acceptable regulatory framework to govern clinical research, enabled research to continue. Opposition to the technology had been overcome through an active process of enrolment and heterogeneous engineering by scientists and public policy makers and the first elements of a socio-technical network around gene therapy had been put in place. During this process gene therapy had been redefined as an experimental medical procedure for the treatment of rare genetic diseases and the direct link with eugenics had been broken. These first elements would later be used by the leading scientific figure in the field, W. French Anderson, to construct a stable network around the development of classical gene therapy. To achieve this, however, he would have to mobilise a wide range of actors and resources to overcome further technical, clinical and political obstacles.

## French Anderson and the organisation of the first clinical trial

French Anderson was one of the earliest advocates of gene therapy. He suggested the possibility of using gene transfer to cure genetic diseases as far back as 1968 (Anonymous 1968) and established the first dedicated gene therapy laboratory in the world in 1974. After spending nearly a decade working on classical gene therapy for thalassemia at NIH, Anderson decided to abandon this line of investigation as a result of technical difficulties, and started a search for a new disease target during 1984 (Anderson 1984).

To achieve this he had to construct what Fujimura has called a 'do-able' research problem (Fujimura 1987), that would be scientifically feasible and at the same time might meet the rigorous criteria being established by the RAC. Anderson wrote a major review of the field and argued that only one disease, adenosine deaminase (ADA) deficiency, might realistically meet these two demands (Anderson 1984). ADA deficiency is a very rare genetic enzyme disorder of the blood that causes a fatal immune deficiency in children. Although less than 30 patients in the US were living with this genetic disease at the time, it had the great advantage that the gene for ADA had recently been isolated.

When he started his work to establish a clinical trial for ADA gene therapy Anderson had few of the resources he needed for a trial: he didn't have a copy of the ADA gene, which was closely guarded by other researchers; and he lacked efficient gene transfer 'vectors'[3] and a means of manufacturing them to the standard required by the Food and Drugs Administration (FDA). Furthermore, he had no access to patients, no experience of managing the disease and was faced by a largely sceptical RAC.

In order to bring together the disparate elements of the network needed to allow his research to proceed Anderson undertook a process of enrolment and heterogeneous engineering. Through the creation of professional alliances he managed to get access to the ADA gene and the gene transfer vectors he needed (Lyon and Gorner 1995). He also teamed-up with Michael Blaese, a clinical researcher specialising in rare immune deficiencies, who provided two ADA patients. The main outstanding problem facing Anderson was the need for manufacturing facilities, the sort of technical support normally provided by industry. However, the production of gene therapy vectors had not been attempted before and no existing firm had either the interest or facilities to undertake this task.

As a consequence, during 1986 Anderson worked with venture capitalists to found the world's first gene therapy firm, Genetic Therapy Inc, with the explicit aim of manufacturing vectors to support a clinical trial of ADA deficiency (Lyon and Gorner 1995). In creating a company Anderson was drawing on the increasingly close association between industry and academia which had arisen during the late 1970s and had become the cornerstone of the emerging biopharmaceutical industry (Wright 1994). It was a mutually beneficial relationship which provided companies with new sources of innovation and scientists with both research funding and potentially lucrative share options and consultancy fees. These academic-industry links were actively encouraged by government policy as a means of increasing industrial competitiveness and a series of legislative initiatives were taken to stimulate technology transfer during this period. In 1986 Congress passed the Federal Technology Transfer Act which enabled government employees to benefit from collaboration with industry, and Anderson established the very first Collaborative Research and Development Agreement (CRADA) under the new law between the NIH and Genetic Therapy Inc.

By 1987 Anderson had put in place almost all the heterogeneous elements of the network, but he still had to win regulatory approval from the RAC. During 1988 he submitted a protocol for the trial and supporting preclinical data, but was refused permission to proceed on the grounds that there was still not enough scientific evidence that the experiment could work. After several months of continuing technical criticism from his scientific peers on the Committee, Anderson made a radical change of tactic and switched to a non-therapeutic gene marking study of cancer using the same basic techniques (Anderson 1993).

The idea of introducing genetic markers to track cells in cancer patients was based on the work of Steven Rosenberg, the President's cancer physician at the time. Blaese and Anderson teamed up with Rosenberg and in 1989 they submitted a protocol to the RAC for an experiment involving the transfer of genetic markers into the white blood cells of patients who had bone marrow transplants to treat leukaemia. After a carefully orchestrated campaign of persuasion and much controversy, the three researchers won the support of a majority of the RAC to vote in favour of this cancer experiment, and in May 1989 the world's first human clinical trial using gene transfer commenced (Lyon and Gorner 1995).

This first trial marked the creation of a stable socio-technical network around somatic gene therapy. Its formation was built on the support won during the ethical debate and the regulatory framework established around the RAC. Two other events were also critical. The first was the link Anderson established with industry, which provided research funding and manufacturing facilities. The second was the switch to cancer which marked a critical turning point in the entire field, as it was the first time that anyone had made a serious proposal for how gene therapy might be applied outside the realm of classical genetic diseases. It was also vital in winning the support of the RAC, cementing the final pieces of the network, and ensuring that all the scientific, social and political resources required for a trial were present. Through this process of enrolment Anderson and Rosenberg articulated a fundamentally new vision for the use of gene therapy and transformed the scope and meaning of gene therapy.

## The gene therapy bandwagon

In the five years following Anderson's landmark trial there was a rapid expansion of the field, both in the USA and internationally, with the number of trials organised in America increasing to over 160 by the end of 1996 (Martin and Thomas 1996). This was accompanied by a dramatic increase in related scientific publications, which rose from under 50 a year in 1989 to over 1,200 in 1996. A large part of this growth was accounted for by the work of other pioneer investigators as they started to organise local socio-technical networks around their own plans for gene therapy trials. As they did this, there was a marked shift in the focus of research away from the classical genetic diseases, which had dominated the field until the eve of the first trial, and towards a range of acquired disorders, most notably cancer. By the end of 1996 over 70 per cent of US trials were for some form of cancer, with less than 10 per cent for genetic diseases (Martin and Thomas 1996).

The construction of local socio-technical networks in many of the leading US medical centres between 1989–93 essentially replicated the structure of the one built around Anderson's trial. Each of these new networks was created by either a clinical researcher or a molecular biologist working in concert with a clinician. In particular, they were constructed around different visions of how gene therapy might be used for the treatment of a given disease and often centred on an attempt to organise a clinical trial. In nearly all cases this also involved starting a new company as a means of getting access to key resources. In the following sections I briefly describe case studies of some of the first attempts to build networks around new applications of the technology. In particular, I pay attention to the way in which the very notion of genetic disease was reconstituted during this process, and how the design for gene therapy technology was fundamentally reshaped as a consequence.

*Gene therapy for genetic diseases*
Following Anderson's first trial a number of different investigators tried to use 'classical' gene therapy as a means of curing a range of very rare genetic disorders. In all cases these trials were based on transferring genes into blood stem cells in order to replace the inherited lack of a particular enzyme. By the end of 1996 a total of seven American trials had been organised and one new firm, Theragen, founded to exploit this technology (Martin and Thomas 1996). However, no stable or long-lasting networks were built around the idea of using classical gene therapy to treat genetic diseases, as it continued to prove impossible to get genes efficiently into blood stem cells. Although all the heterogeneous elements had been configured into local networks to support these trials, they ultimately fell apart due to the recalcitrance of nature. As a consequence, most researchers abandoned the classical approach that had provided the basis for the first trial

and dominated the field until 1990, and started looking for ways of delivering genes to other cell types.

Despite the failure of classical gene therapy, the possibility of treating other genetic diseases attracted scientific and commercial interest during the 1990s. In 1989 Ron Crystal, a leading chest physician at the NIH, suggested that it might be possible to transfer genes into the lungs (Rosenfeld *et al.* 1991) and within two years the main clinical target for this strategy was established as cystic fibrosis (CF), the most common genetic disorder in Caucasians. However, it was felt that a permanent cure for CF would not be possible because of the difficulty in transplanting cells into the lining of the lung. Instead, the therapy would have to be applied in vivo, and involved spraying vectors containing the therapeutic gene directly into the lung airway. It would therefore need to be repeated every few months and would act in a similar manner to a conventional drug.

Three different groups of researchers were successful in getting RAC approval for human trials of this strategy in 1992. To help organise their trials, each either started a new gene therapy firm or collaborated with an established company: Ron Crystal founded GenVec, Jim Wilson started Genovo and Michael Welsh formed a close working relationship with Genzyme, a large biotechnology firm (Martin 1998). By the end of 1996 a total of 13 clinical trials for CF had been approved by the RAC, each network embodying the idea of using gene therapy as a form of drug delivery to treat a lung disease.

*Gene therapy for cancer*
The first gene marking study organised by Rosenberg, Blaese and Anderson established the principle of using human gene transfer to treat cancer and this prospect was quickly explored by a number of other investigators. By the end of 1996 over 25 gene marking and 88 gene therapy trials for the disease had been approved by the RAC (Martin and Thomas 1996). The majority of these trials simply integrated gene transfer techniques into existing strategies for immunotherapy and chemotherapy, enabling the rapid diffusion of the technology throughout the already well established networks supporting cancer research.

In addition to the ease with which it fitted into existing patterns of experimental practice, a major factor enabling the development of gene therapy in this area was the changing conception of cancer. Increasingly, the disease was being constructed as essentially genetic in origin (Fujimura 1996). By the early 1990s scientists believed that tumours were often formed by the inactivation of tumour suppressor genes which regulated the normal growth of a cell. If these genes were turned off, as a result of damage caused by say smoking, the cell would divide in an uncontrolled fashion leading to a tumour. Although such an explanation did not evoke a genetic explanation based on heredity, this new molecular pathology offered the possibility of describing cancer in terms of the regulation and control of particular genes.

For the advocates of gene therapy, if a diagnosis could be made in molecular terms, then it might also be possible to intervene therapeutically at this level using gene transfer.

This approach to gene therapy was in essence a form of in vivo gene replacement and was first advocated by Friedmann and Lee who envisaged delivering tumour suppressor genes to cancers as a means of inhibiting their growth (Huang et al. 1988). Impetus was given to this strategy in the late 1980s by work in gene sequencing which led to the identification of a number of tumour suppressor genes. However, the strategy was only put into practice in 1992 by Jack Roth, a cancer surgeon, when he gained RAC approval for a clinical trial involving the direct administration of the P53 tumour suppressor gene in patients suffering from lung cancer (Roth et al. 1994). In order to get access to both the financial resources and vector technology required to start a trial, Roth founded the firm Introgen with the aim of commercially developing P53 therapy (Jack Roth, personal communication). In organising this trial and founding his company Roth embodied the notion that cancer was a genetic disease in both the local socio-technical network and the very design of the therapy itself. Without the central idea that cancer could be thought of as a genetic disease this therapy would not have come about.

*Cell implants—gene therapy to deliver drugs*
In the light of the problems of getting genes into blood stem cells, by the late 1980s researchers were starting to investigate the possibility of transferring genes into a wide range of other tissues, including the skin, the liver, the brain and the heart. At the same time a new therapeutic concept started to emerge whereby genes might be used as a means of locally producing therapeutic proteins.[4] For example, if a patient's cells could be removed, genetically modified ex vivo to contain the gene for Factor VIII, and then reimplanted at a suitable location, they might be able to secrete this missing blood clotting protein into the blood stream as a means of treating haemophilia. In principle, these cell implants would function like mechanical drug delivery devices. This new vision for gene therapy was a radical break with the previously dominant idea of treating relatively rare genetic diseases, as it reconceptualised the technology so that it might be used to treat other more common acquired conditions.

One of the first researchers to pursue this strategy was Richard Selden, who suggested that a patient's own skin cells could be genetically modified to secrete insulin as a cure for diabetes (Selden et al. 1987). In a related proposal, Fred Gage and Theodore Friedmann, planned to genetically modify skin cells to secrete a protein, Nerve Growth Factor (NGF), and then reimplant them in the brain as a way of treating Alzheimer's disease (Gage et al. 1987). Other proposals were made for the use of a range of different cell types: Woo and Ledley suggested using modified liver cells as a means treating haemophilia (Ledley et al. 1987); and Mulligan and Nabel independently envisaged using cell implants to reduce cholesterol levels in chronic heart disease (Wilson *et al.* 1989, Nabel *et al.* 1989).

In each of these cases the development of novel therapeutic strategies was only possible as a result of the researchers being able to describe the pathology terms of molecular genetics. In some cases, such as haemophilia, the primary cause of the disease was clearly inherited, but as with cancer, it was also possible to construct a model of these other acquired conditions in terms of problems in the way the gene was regulated in the body. For example, Alzheimer's might be caused by the production of too little nerve growth factor (NGF) in the brain as a result of damage to the NGF gene. The role of gene therapy in these cases was therefore to restore the level of the missing protein coded by the damaged gene. This shift to a 'molecular pathology' was enabled by progress in many areas of biology, in particular, the information coming from gene sequencing and the recently formed Human Genome Project. By the early 1990s it was becoming possible to describe many diseases in purely molecular terms, with the prospect of all pathologies eventually being categorised in this way.

The three main groups of researchers working on cell implants led by Mulligan, Selden, and Friedmann and Gage each set about creating sociotechnical networks around their particular visions of the technology in order to get access to the resources required to sustain their research. In particular, they all formed companies with the intention of moving their therapies into human trials (Martin 1998). See Table 1 for details.

However, by the mid 1990s the notion of using cell implants was starting to be abandoned by the field in favour of direct in vivo therapeutic strategies which could be more easily incorporated into existing patterns of clinical practice, were less technically demanding and, above all, more commercially attractive. As with gene therapy for cystic fibrosis, many of these approaches were conceptualised in a similar fashion to conventional drugs. In this vision, gene therapies would be designed to act over relatively short periods of time rather than providing a permanent cure, would be mass-produced and administered by conventional means such as a simple injection. By 1992 George Wu had established TargeTech to pursue the idea of developing 'gene Drugs' for haemophilia and heart disease. In the following year Fred Ledley and Savio Woo founded GeneMedicine to investigate in vivo therapies for liver disorders and emphysema (Martin 1998).

A significant factor in the development of gene therapy as a form of in vivo drug delivery was the entry of the pharmaceutical industry into the emerging socio-technical network. In the early history of the technology the major pharmaceutical companies had been largely uninvolved, but in 1993–94 a wave of alliances and acquisitions was created with the nascent gene therapy industry. By 1996 over $1 billion of investment had been committed by the pharmaceutical industry to small gene therapy firms, most of

Table 1: *Scientific pioneers and the Founding of Dedicated Gene Therapy Firms*

| Firm | Scientific founders | Date founded | Disease | Initial clinical strategy | |
|---|---|---|---|---|---|
| | | | | Mode | Strategy |
| Genetic Therapy | Anderson | 1986/7 | ADA deficiency | ex vivo | transfer to blood stem cells |
| Viagene | Jolly | 1987 | HIV/cancer | ex/in vivo | therapeutic vaccines |
| Somatix | Mulligan | 1987/8 | Dwarfism | ex vivo | cell implants |
| | | | Diabetes | | |
| TransKaryotic Therapies | Selden | 1988 | Haemophilia | ex vivo | cell implants |
| | | | Dwarfism | | |
| Targeted Genetics | Greenberg Miller | 1989 | HIV | ex vivo | transfer to blood stem cells |
| TargeTech | Wu | 1989 | Haemophilia | in vivo | transfer to liver |
| Vical | Wolff | 1990 | Infections | in vivo | vaccines |
| | Nabel | | Cancer | in vivo | immunotherapy |
| GeneSys | Friedmann Gage | 1990 | Parkinson's disease | ex vivo | cell implants |
| Canji | Lee | 1990 | Cancer | in vivo | tumour suppressors |
| Theragen | Barranger Glorioso | 1991 | Gaucher's disease | ex vivo | transfer to blood stem cells |
| Genovo | Wilson | 1992 | Cystic fibrosis | ex vivo | transfer to lung |
| GeneMedicine | Ledley Woo | 1993 | Emphysema | in vivo | transfer to lung |
| Introgen | Roth | 1993 | Cancer | in vivo | tumour suppressor |
| GenVec | Crystal | 1993 | Cystic fibrosis | in vivo | transfer to lung |

it going to support the further development of these in vivo therapies (Martin 1998). A major reason for this interest was that the construction of gene therapy as a drug fitted easily into the dominant pharmaceutical product paradigm and was much more attractive to large firms than therapies based on classical gene therapy or ex vivo cell implants. The very heavy investment made in this area fundamentally shifted the locus of power in the network and the focus of research, reinforcing the shift to using genes as drugs.

Although the pioneers of cell implants were ultimately unsuccessful in attracting enough support to form long-lasting socio-technical networks, the strategy marked a decisive break from classical gene therapy. In particular, it opened up the possibility of using gene transfer technology for the treatment of many common acquired conditions. It also paved the way for the subsequent shift to direct in vivo therapies and the move from permanent to transient cures.

In the years following the initial trials described above, gene transfer was applied to virtually every tissue and organ in the body, and therapeutic strategies were developed for a wide range of other common acquired diseases including AIDS, arthritis and heart disease (Martin and Thomas 1996). Table 2 shows the full range of human diseases which gene therapy was being experimentally applied to, in either model systems or human trials, by 1996, and includes many major chronic conditions. A series of other socio-technical networks and companies were created during the 1990s to support these new applications and details of the most important ones are given in Table 1. However, it must be stressed that despite this rapid expansion in clinical interest, the field remained essentially experimental, with no working therapy at the end of 1999.

The application of gene therapy to such a broad range of diseases prompted some advocates to see it as a potential new therapeutic modality, which could in principle be used to tackle virtually any pathology (Crystal 1995). Furthermore, the development of the technology by this stage was no longer wedded to the ideas of classical genetics, but was instead guided by the new therapeutic opportunities created by describing common acquired diseases in the language of molecular genetics.

## Conclusion

The case studies described above illustrate the utility of using concepts from the sociology of technology to investigate the way in which new knowledge, and new disease concepts are co-constructed during the process of technological innovation. This chapter has also shown that the development of gene therapy simultaneously required a series of technical, cognitive and social changes. For pioneering investigators to apply gene therapy to research problems in specific clinical niches, they had to engage in a process

Table 2: *Diseases Targeted by Research into Human Gene Therapy in 1996*

| Genetic diseases | Cancers | Cardiovascular disease | Viral diseases | Neurological disorders | Other chronic conditions | Other conditions |
|---|---|---|---|---|---|---|
| ADA/SCID | Many types of cancer, including: | Atherosclerosis | HIV | Parkinson's | Arthritis | Wound healing |
| PNP deficiency | | Peripheral vascular disease | CMV | Alzheimer's | Lupus | Burns |
| Gaucher's disease | | | Immunisation | | Diabetes | Dental problems |
| Lesch-Nyhan syndrome | – leukaemia | Restenosis | against many | | Liver diseases | Baldness |
| PKU deficiency | – breast | | others | | Emphysema | |
| Pituitary dwarfism | – ovarian | | including: | | Skin ulcers | |
| Cystic fibrosis | – skin | | – hepatitis | | Kidney disease | |
| Duchenne Muscular Dystrophy | – lung | | – herpes | | Eye diseases | |
| Familial hypercholesterolemia | – kidney | | – influenza | | | |
| Thalassemia | – brain | | | | | |
| Haemophilia A & B | – colon | | | | | |

of heterogeneous socio-technical engineering (Callon 1987). This included, the re-conceptualisation of particular diseases as being genetic in some way; the reshaping of the technology itself; the construction of local socio-technical networks of regulators, genes, firms, clinicians and patients; and the creation of a new industry. The hybrid theoretical framework outlined in the introduction has provided a useful means for analysing these events and demonstrates that it is possible to describe the process of innovation and technical change in sociological terms.

It has been shown that the application of gene therapy to a broad range of common acquired conditions has reconceptualised them within the language of molecular genetics. At the same time, the very idea of a genetic disease was itself reconstructed so that it was no longer restricted to inherited disorders, but included cancer, heart disease and many other acquired conditions. Through this process it became possible to describe a given pathology as being acquired and operating at a genetic level. The point is well illustrated by the example of cancer, where the dominant model of this acquired disease started to become genetic in the early 1990s. This led to the introduction of novel anti-cancer strategies based on gene replacement and the development of these new gene therapies in turn further strengthened the notion that cancer was caused by errors in the way genes worked.

Through the development of this molecular pathology a new type of genetic body has been constructed in which all biological functions can be described in the language of genetics (Turney and Balmer 1998). This cognitive change has been embodied in new therapeutic technologies, new forms of clinical practice and a new industry, and was enabled by the new knowledge flowing from the Human Genome Project.

The chapter has also demonstrated that this reconception of genetic disease has both depended on, and enabled, a major change in the definition, applications and design of gene therapy technology itself. During the 30 years between the first proposal for genetic therapy and the growth of clinical applications in the 1990s, gene therapy technology was fundamentally reshaped as attempts were made to design a technology around which stable networks might be built. It moved from being a largely surgical procedure for the treatment of rare inherited disorders to a novel form of drug therapy for cancer and other acquired diseases.

In particular, four major changes in the design of the technology occurred as it moved from being a scientific idea to a clinical reality. Firstly, the link to eugenics was broken when germ line therapy was ruled unethical, paving the way for the legitimate development of somatic therapy. The second change was the break with classical genetics that occurred when the first cancer trial was approved and classical gene therapy, for technical reasons, was abandoned as a serious option. This opened up the possibility of treating a wide range of acquired diseases through the development of cell implants. Following this, the next major transition was marked by the shift from gene therapy as an ex vivo surgical procedure to it becoming a form of in vivo drug delivery. Simultaneously, the technology was reconfigured to provide a temporary rather than a permanent cure.

Each of these transformations in the application and physical design of gene therapy occurred as investigators struggled to build stable networks and each involved the reconstitution of the concept of genetic disease. Only by reshaping the technology and redefining genetic disease in this manner was it ultimately possible to enrol all the groups and resources required to introduce gene therapy into the clinic. In this sense the technology, the process of network formation and the changing concept of what a genetic disease was, mutually shaped each other. Central to this process of network building was the creation of particular visions for how gene therapy might be applied to treat a given disease and these were used as a means of both enrolling support and guiding research (van Lente 1993).

Finally, a key issue this chapter has highlighted was the role of corporate firms in both enabling the development of gene therapy and in shaping the direction of research. In particular, the formation of the biotechnology industry during the 1980s, and the common financial interests amongst scientists and companies resulting from this, was fundamental to the growth of the field. Dedicated gene therapy firms were created by researchers as both a means of exploiting research for profit and a mechanism for gaining access to a range of heterogeneous financial, technical and managerial resources. The entry of pharmaceutical companies into the network in 1993 increased the power of firms to influence the technology and helped transform gene therapy into an experimental form of drug therapy for the treatment of a wide range of acquired diseases.

## Notes

1   It should be noted that the distinction between these two options was not always clearcut, with scientists such as W. French Anderson advocating the genetic modification of future generations for purely medical purposes, a position he continued to maintain during the 1990s. However, a clear distinction was made between these two concepts during the 1960s by scientific advocates of genetic therapy (Tatum 1966, see Martin 1998 for discussion).

2   The ideas of classical genetics were first applied to medicine by the British physician Archibald Garrod, who in his book *Inborn Factors of Disease* published in 1931, suggested a simple correlation between inherited factors and particular familial conditions (Schriver and Childs 1989).

3   The term vector refers to the mechanism by which genes are transferred into the target cell. Prior to 1990 this mainly involved the use of genetically modified viruses which were engineered to incorporate the therapeutic gene.

4   The terms therapeutic protein or protein drug simply refer to the protein which is produced in the body by the introduction of the therapeutic gene.

# References

Anderson, W.F. (1984) Prospects for human gene therapy, *Science*, 226, 401–9.

Anderson, W.F. (1993) Musings on the struggle—Part III: the October 3 RAC Meeting, *Human Gene Therapy*, 4, 401–2.

Anonymous (1968) Repair of genetic defects predicted, *Pediatric News*, 2, 6, 28–9.

Berg, M. (1997) *Rationalizing Medical Work: Decision-Support Techniques and Medical Practice*. Cambridge, MA: MIT Press.

Bijker, W.E. (1995) *Of Bicycles, Bakelites and Bulbs: Towards a Theory of Sociotechnical Change*. Cambridge, MA: MIT Press.

Bijker, W.E., Hughes, T.P. and Pinch, T.J. (eds) (1987) *The Social Construction of Technological Systems*. Cambridge, MA: MIT Press.

Blume, S.S. (1992) *Insight and Industry: on the Dynamics of Technological Change in Medicine*. Cambridge, MA: MIT Press.

Callon, M. (1987) Society in the making: the study of technology as a tool for sociological analysis. In Bijker, W.E., Hughes, T.P. and Pinch, T.J. (eds) *The Social Construction of Technological Systems*. Cambridge, MA: MIT Press.

Capron, A.M. (1990) The impact of the report *Splicing Life, Human Gene Therapy*, 1, 1, 69–71.

Clarke, A. and Montini, T. (1993) The many faces of RU486: tales of situated knowledges and technological contestations, *Science, Technology and Human Values*, 18, 1, 42–78.

Cook-Deegan, R.M. (1990) Human gene therapy and Congress, *Human Gene Therapy*, 1, 163–70.

Crystal, R. (1995) Transfer of genes into humans: early lessons and obstacles to success, *Science*, 270, 404–10.

Elston, M.A. (ed) (1997) *The Sociology of Medical Science and Technology*. Oxford: Blackwell Publishers.

Fujimura, J. (1987) Constructing do-able problems in cancer research: articulating alignment, *Social Studies of Science*, 17, 257–93.

Fujimura, J.H. (1996) *Crafting Science: a Sociohistory of the Quest for the Genetics of Cancer*. Cambridge, MA: Harvard University Press.

Gage, F.H., Wolff, J.A., Rosenberg, M.B., Xu, L., Yee, J-K., Shults, C. and Friedmann, T. (1987) Grafting genetically modified cells to the brain: possibilities for the future, *Neuroscience*, 23, 795–807.

Haldane, J.B.S. (1923) *Daedalus* or science and the future. In Dronamraju, K.R. (ed) *Haldane's Daedalus Revisited*. Oxford: Oxford University Press.

Hotchkiss, R.D. (1965) Potential for a genetic engineering, *Journal of Heredity*, 56, 197.

Huang, H.J.S., Yee, J-K., Shew, J-K., Chen, P-L., Bookstein, R., Friedmann, T., Lee, E. and Lee, W-H. (1988) Suppression of the neoplastic phenotype by replacement of the RB gene in human cancer cells, *Science*, 242, 1563–6.

Hughes, T.P. (1987) The evolution of large technical systems. In Bijker, W.E., Hughes, T.P. and Pinch, T.J. (eds) *The Social Construction of Technological Systems*. Cambridge, MA: MIT Press.

Kay, L.E. (1993) *The Molecular Vision of Life: Caltech, the Rockefeller Foundation, and the Rise of the New Biology*. Oxford: Oxford University Press.

Kevles, D.J. (1985) *In the Name of Eugenics*. Harmondsworth: Penguin Books.

Kevles, D.J. (1992) Out of eugenics: the historical politics of the Human Genome

Project. In Kevles, D.J. and Hood, L. (eds) *The Code of Codes*. Cambridge, MA: Harvard University Press.

Koch, L. (1993) *The Genetification of Medicine and the Concept of Disease*. Diskussionspapier, 1–9. Hamburg: Hamburger Institut für Sozialforschung.

Koch, L. and Stemerding, D. (1994) The sociology of entrenchment: a cystic fibrosis test for everyone, *Social Science and Medicine*, 39, 9, 1211–20.

Lawrence, C. (1997) 'Definite and material': coronary thrombosis and cardiologists in the 1920s. In Rosenberg, C.E. and Golden, J. (eds) *Framing Disease: Studies in Cultural History*. New Brunswick, NJ: Rutgers University Press.

Ledley, F.D., Darlington, G.J., Hahn, T. and Woo, S.L. (1987) Retroviral gene transfer into primary hepatocytes: implications for genetic therapy of liver-specific functions, *Proceedings of the National Academy of Sciences*, 84, 5335–9.

Luria, S.E. (1969) Modern biology: a terrifying power, *Nation*, 20 October, 406.

Lyon, J. and Gorner, P. (1995) *Altered Fates: Gene Therapy and the Retooling of Human Life*. New York: Norton and Company.

MacKenzie, D. and Wajcman, J. (1985) *The Social Shaping of Technology*. Milton Keynes: Open University Press.

Martin, P.A. (1998) *From Eugenics to Therapeutics: Science and the Reshaping of Gene Therapy Technology*. Unpublished DPhil Thesis. Brighton: University of Sussex.

Martin, P.A. and Thomas, S.M. (1996) *The Development of Gene Therapy in Europe and the United States: a Comparative Analysis*. STEEP Special Report No. 5. Brighton: Science Policy Research Unit, University of Sussex.

Muller, H.J. (1935) *Out of the Night; a Biologist's View of the Future*. New York: Vanguard Press.

Muller, H. (1965) Means and aims in human genetic betterment. In Sonneborn, T.M. (ed) *The Control of Human Heredity and Evolution*. New York: Macmillan.

Nabel, E.M., Plautz, G., Boyce, F.M., Stanley, J.C. and Nabel, G.J. (1989) Recombinant gene expression *in vivo* within endothelial cells of the arterial wall, *Science*, 244, 1342–4.

National Institutes of Health (1985) Points to consider in the design and submission of human somatic-cell gene therapy protocols, *Federal Register*, 50, 33463–7.

Oudshoorn, N. (1994) *Beyond the Natural Body: an Archaeology of Sex Hormones*. London: Routledge.

Palmiter, R.D., Brinster, R.L. and Hammer, R.E. (1982) Dramatic growth of mice that develop from eggs microinjected with metallothionein-growth hormone fusion gene, *Nature*, 300, 611–15.

Pauly, P.J. (1987) *Controlling Life: Jacques Loeb and the Engineering Ideal in Biology*. New York: Oxford University Press.

Peitzman, S.J. (1997) From Bright's disease to end-stage renal disease. In Rosenberg, C.E. and Golden, J. (eds) *Framing Disease: Studies in Cultural History*. New Brunswick, NJ: Rutgers University Press.

Pinch, T.J. and Bijker, W.E. (1984) The social construction of facts and artifacts—or how the sociology of science and the sociology of technology might benefit each other, *Social Studies of Science*, 14, 3, 399–441.

President's Commission for the Study of Ethical Problems in Medicine and Biomedical and Behavioural Research (1982) *Splicing Life: the Social and Ethical Issues of Genetic Engineering with Human Beings*. Washington DC: US Government Printing Office.

Prout, A. (1996) Actor-network theory, technology and medical sociology: an illustrative example of the metered dose inhaler, *Sociology of Health and Illness*, 18, 2, 198–219.

Rosenberg, C.E. and Golden, J. (eds) (1997) *Framing Disease: Studies in Cultural History*. New Brunswick, NJ: Rutgers University Press.

Rosenfeld, M.A., Siegfried, W., Yoshimura, K., Fukayama, M., Stier, L.E., Paakko, P.K., Gilardi, P., Stratford-Pericaudet, L.D., Pericaudet, M. and Crystal, R. (1991) Adenovirus mediated transfer of a recombinant alpha-1-antitrypsin gene to the lung epithelium in vivo, *Science*, 252, 431–4.

Roth, J., Mukhopadhyay, T., Zhang, W.W., Fujiwara, T. and Georges, R. (1994) Gene replacement strategies for the prevention and therapy of cancer, *European Journal of Cancer*, 30A, 13, 2032–7.

Saetnan, A.R. (1991) Rigid politics and technological flexibility—the anatomy of a failed hospital innovation, *Science, Technology and Human Values*, 16, 4, 419–47.

Scriver, C.R. and Childs, B. (eds) (1989) *Garrod's Inborn Factors in Disease*. Oxford: Oxford University Press.

Selden, R., Skoskiewicz, M.J., Howie, K.B., Russell, P.S. and Goodman, H.M. (1987) Implantation of genetically engineered fibroblasts into mice: implications for gene therapy, *Science*, 236, 714–18.

Stapledon, W.O. (1930) *Last and First Men*. London: Methuen.

Szybalski, W. (1992) Use of the HPRT gene and the HAT selection technique in DNA-mediated transformation of mammalian cells: first steps toward developing hybidoma techniques and gene therapy, *Bioessays*, 14, 7, 495–500.

Tatum, E.L. (1958) A case history in biomedical research. In *Nobel Lectures in Molecular Biology 1933–1975*. New York: Elsevier.

Tatum, E.L. (1966) Molecular biology, nucleic acids and the future of medicine, *Perspectives in Biology and Medicine*, Autumn, 19–32.

Turney, J. (1998) *Frankenstein's Footsteps: Science, Genetics and Popular Culture*. New Haven: Yale University Press.

Turney, J. and Balmer, B. (1998) The genetic body. In Pickstone, J. (ed) *Medicine in the Twentieth Century*. Manchester: Manchester University Press.

van Lente, H. (1993) *Promising Technology: the Dynamics of Expectations in Technological Developments*. Enschede: University of Twente.

Wailoo, K. (1997) *Drawing Blood: Technology and Disease Identity in Twentieth-Century America*. Baltimore: Johns Hopkins University Press.

Wilson, J.M., Birinyi, L.K., Salomon, R.N., Libby, P., Xallows, A.D. and Mulligan, R.C. (1989) Implantation of vascular grafts lined with genetically modified endothelial cells, *Science*, 244, 1344–7.

Wright, P. and Treacher, A. (eds) (1982) *The Problem of Medical Knowledge*. Edinburgh: Edinburgh University Press.

Wright, S. (1994) *Molecular Politics: Developing American and British Regulatory Policy for Genetic Engineering, 1972–1982*. Chicago: The University of Chicago Press.

# 2. Experts as 'storytellers' in reproductive genetics: exploring key issues

## Elizabeth Ettorre

### Introduction

The culture of medicine and specifically, the professional practices of physicians concerning childbirth and childbearing have changed dramatically with rapid technological developments, especially those generated by geneticists (Steinberg 1997). As experts tell us that a greater proportion of childhood disease is genetic in origin, the contribution of genetic factors to a whole range of diseases becomes socially visible (Clarke 1997: 5). Shaped by an understanding of the impact of biotechnology on medical practice, this chapter focuses on reproductive genetics, defined as the utilisation of DNA-based technologies in the medical management and supervision of reproduction. Although this concept, reproductive genetics, may appear, at first glance, as biomedical, it is not. Reproductive genetics is a sociological concept employed to demonstrate that powerful social and cultural processes are involved in the organisation of genetic tests for prenatal diagnosis, already identified as an intricate sociotechnological system (Cowan 1994: 35).

In feminist contexts, this concept, reproductive genetics, has been used to demonstrate that it is not possible to treat women and men in the same way with regard to reproduction (Mahowald 1994: 69), and that it is on this wider social plane that the moral stakes are highest (Faden 1994: 88). In a related feminist context, Shildrick (1997: 22) contends that the long process of conception and gestation is internal to the female body, and that the reproductive body stands for something essentially female. Wendell (1992: 71) argues further that reproductive genetics represents one of the most successful achievements of modern medicine to control 'nature'. In her view, reproductive genetics is a powerful strategy within the Western scientific project to idealise the 'perfect' body and thus shape contemporary conceptions of able-bodiness and disability.

With the development of reproductive genetics, prenatal technologies are used increasingly for fetal diagnosis. The procedures can be either non-DNA based (*i.e.* not directly related to genetics—such as ultrasound scanning) or DNA-based (*i.e.* related to genetics and blood or serum collection—such as chorionic villus screening, maternal serum screening or amniocentesis). Prenatal screening is a complicated social process which involves numerous tests, myriad relations with a variety of medical personnel (*e.g.* obstetricians, genetic counsellors, midwives, pediatricians) and complex decision making processes, extending, in some cases, over several pregnancies (Parsons and Atkinson 1993).

Prenatal screening of fetuses for congenital conditions (*i.e.* fetal diagnosis) allows physicians to perform selective abortion of 'affected' fetuses. For them, a specific genetic technique may appear as one of many solutions to the problems that modern reproductive medicine seeks to solve. For example, physicians, especially obstetricians, want to manage, treat and help their patients, pregnant women, to deliver healthy babies. In their expert view, maternal serum screening, chorionic villus screening or amniocentesis are techniques which allow this to happen. Nevertheless, some pregnant women may experience devastating consequences in their encounters with these techniques (Tymstra 1991, Rothman 1994).

In many countries today, medical experts (Asch *et al.* 1996, Beekhuis 1993, Brock *et al.* 1996, Heinonen *et al.* 1996, Mantingh *et al.* 1991, Wald *et al.* 1995, Wald *et al.* 1996) contend that most, if not all, pregnant women should undergo prenatal diagnosis and be screened for genetic disorders. At the same time, men and women in the general population believe that these sorts of techniques can be useful in eliminating a variety of serious diseases (Marteau 1995). As social trends in the public's perception of reproductive genetics materialise, important questions are being raised (Ettorre 1997). What genetic diseases will be perceived as serious or life-threatening? Along with cystic fibrosis and Huntington's disease, will alcoholism, homosexuality, schizophrenia be included in the list of these diseases? What about poverty or unemployment? Will a hierarchy of social diseases be created and used as a basis for discrimination? If so, who will decide on this hierarchy? Is there an already 'invisible hierarchy' developing from the use of prenatal diagnostic techniques? How do these techniques affect women to whom in the main they are applied? Answers to the above questions are beyond the scope of this chapter. Nevertheless, they suggest that there is a need for substantive, empirical work on the impact of reproductive genetics upon society, and scope for theoretical elaborations on how 'the social construction of 'biological phenomenon' (Lippmann 1994a) has become embedded in contemporary culture.

In the light of the above, the main aim of this chapter is to report on findings from a European study on experts' perceptions of reproductive genetics and to explore the notion of experts as 'genetic story tellers' and producers of genetic ideology. After discussing methods, I turn in the first part of the chapter to: (1) examine the notion of experts as genetic story tellers; and (2) provide experts' accounts of families who are perceived as being in need of prenatal genetic screening. In this part I look at the types of claims being constructed by genetic story tellers as well as the impact of these claims. The second part of the chapter is a theoretical elaboration of how, in making their claims, experts employ a series of normative strategies in the cultural production of genetics work.

## Methods

### The sample

The source of empirical data presented in this chapter is a qualitative study on experts' accounts of the use of prenatal genetic screening in four European countries: the UK, Finland, the Netherlands and Greece. This study is part of a series of comparative studies in this area, being conducted by a European consortium of researchers. For the experts' study, the initial number of interviews was set at 10 in each country and the goal was to interview equal numbers of geneticists, clinicians, practitioners, lawyers and/or ethicists, policy makers, public health officials and researchers in each country. While the study focus was on biomedical not lay experts, this is not meant to imply that only professionals can be experts, a view that can be disputed (Calnan 1987, Davison *et al.* 1991). Given that the aim of the study was to review the role of key players influential in public debates in each country, every effort was made to find experts who were active in this area either clinically or academically. It was decided that one person, the Project Co-ordinator (author), would carry out all of the expert interviews.

### Data collection and analysis

In each country, experts were selected, contacted and asked whether or not they would be interested in providing their views. The initial liaison work was done by the research partners. The author set dates when she would be visiting each country and arranged times and places for the interviews. Between October 1995 and December 1996, it was planned to interview 40 experts from each country. In practice, although it was possible to reach the desired number of 10 interviews in Finland and Greece, this was not possible in the Netherlands and the UK, in each of which nine interviews were undertaken. This was due mainly to the study timetable and budget. All interviews needed to be completed by December 1996, and the researcher had one week's time to interview experts in each country. To supplement these 38 interviews, 'unofficial' interviews (*i.e.* without the use of a tape recorder) were carried out: four in the Netherlands and three in the UK. These interviews were mainly with postgraduate medical students or biomedical researchers with expertise in the area. The data obtained from these unofficial interviews were not used in the data analyses and were perceived by the author as providing background information in specific countries.

Experts were asked their views on genetic testing and screening in prenatal diagnosis. The interview questions revolved around their attitudes on the use of these techniques; their perceptions of the prevailing state of knowledge on legal, medical and ethical aspects; social effects; and policy priorities at local and national levels. The interviews were tape recorded and lasted between 30 and 90 minutes: the average was an hour. All interview data were transcribed and themes were identified by Word Perfect (Windows) Quick Finder Index.

These themes were discussed amongst the research partners. Excerpts from these interviews will be used in this chapter.

Some variations of experts' attitudes occurred within specific disciplines (*e.g.* clinical geneticists disagreed with other clinical geneticists), amongst disciplines (*e.g.* differences between clinical geneticists, obstetricians, ethicists, policy makers) and between countries (*e.g.* differences between Dutch and UK experts). It is beyond the scope of this chapter to discuss these issues in detail, and reporting on these variations has been, or is currently being, undertaken in other contexts (Ettorre 1996, Ettorre *et al.* 1997, Ettorre *et al.* 1999). In this chapter, the focus is mainly on similarities in experts' perceptions and attitudes as a group, but some variations emerge in the latter half of the chapter.

## Experts as 'genetic story tellers'

Barbara Katz Rothman has argued that genetics isn't just a science: it is a way of thinking—'an ideology for our time' (1998a: 18). She contends that scientists constantly make decisions about what they consider significant and that their choices reflect the society in which they live and work. For Rothman, scientists are not detached observers of nature: they produce culture. In a similar vein of thought, Lippman constructs a view of biomedical experts as the primary 'story tellers'—the whole range of professionals that have a 'wealth of raw material from which to choose when they construct their explanations, their stories, for the conditions that interest them' (1994b: 12). While she likens scientists to novelists and contends that both sets of authors shape and explain their raw material to convey messages reducing their complexities in order to 'tell a story', she suggests that these stories reflect their personal views and the prevailing social and cultural context (1994b: 12). For Lippmann, 'all citizens of the world' are the audience for genetics storytellers (1992: 1469). Given this vast scope, these storytellers attempt to construct complex genetic narratives accessible for popular consumption in both the popular and professional media. This is an important, if not the most important, part of 'genetics work', establishing their scientific and cultural authority by the stories scientists tell, the metaphors they use (Rosner and Johnson 1995) and the global range of their influence.

In this context, Duster contends that while experts work within the prism of heritability, how this genetic prism refracts and thereby selects problems for research, screening and treatment is a matter for the sociology of knowledge (1990: 18). He argues that at specific points in time, particular, social questions emerge for detailed inspection and set the path for the prevailing epistemology of a culture. In his view, today's path is science under the banner of the new genetics. Duster insists further that while experts say that the new genetics will bring greater health to various groups in society, their approach does not address effectively the 'truth' claims of genetics—claims that are shaped by the workings of contemporary science and the cultural need for genetics. For example, in making truth claims, experts establish 'scientific proof' through particular lines of enquiry or paths of knowledge (1990: 21). By setting up research programmes and influencing public policy, they legitimate their authority. On the other hand, their claims are shaped by the concerns of a culture in which there is an increased role for the explanatory basis of genetics in an array of behaviours and conditions (Duster 1990: 94)—what Lippman (1994b) calls geneticisation.

Here, Duster believes that any scientific advancements, promises or problems, applied to populations will inevitably imply a certain amount of unease, especially for populations at risk. In this context, Higgs argues that pregnant women, one such 'population at risk', may feel unease, given that many of their own life experiences are being taken over by a detached medical elite (1997: 163). Pregnant women's unease at the direction taken by modern medicine can become problematic for them, particularly if it is combined with 'manufactured uncertainty' (Giddens 1991): the result of too much information about risks and no way of assessing the impact of these risks. One such example is the controversy over the need for amniocentesis against its potential for causing miscarriages, psychological disturbance or what Rothman (1994) terms 'tentative pregnancies'.

In the above discussion, I have explored the notion of experts as genetic story tellers. Next, I will examine experts' accounts of families who are perceived as being in need of prenatal genetic screening as well as the types of claims that experts construct, and the impact of these claims.

### Experts, 'normal patient families' and reproductive genetics

A shared perception concerning the sorts of families, deemed appropriate to treat 'genetically' emerged in experts' accounts. This perception involved distinguishing between patients who were 'normal' (*i.e.* without genetic problems and therefore outside the domain of genetics) and those who were 'normal patients' (*i.e.* families with a genetics problem). For example, a clinical geneticist stated:

> Most people working in this field see a distinction here [*i.e.* between families] . . . We don't see the sort of normal people . . . We see the normal, patient family . . . a family with a genetic problem. . . . I think [they] will always be there, they will always need genetic counselling and they will want genetic testing for a defined problem that is known in that family. (A17).[1]

The above statement confirms Richards' contention that patients are 'now families, not individuals' (1993: 578). Thus, the effect of seeing a geneticist is a family issue with implications for several members, as the following excerpt illustrates:

> [Genetic data] are shared by your siblings, parents, sisters and brothers
> . . . What [they] find in you does not just concern you, it concerns the
> whole family. It makes the situation much more different than if it was
> just your own (A4 clinical geneticist).

Powerful concepts such as 'risk', 'affected offspring', 'viability', 'defective genes' and 'carrier status', along with all sorts of technologies (*e.g.* amniocentesis, maternal serum screening, CVS, genetic testing) are mobilised by experts in describing 'bodies in families' with genetic problems. When a family undergoes genetic testing, this experience tends to dominate the whole course of a pregnancy. The terms, 'carrier status' and 'risk', take on new meanings, as families attempt to balance the relationship between how experts perceive their levels of 'risk' and the family's own perceived levels of 'risk' (Parson and Atkinson 1993). One consequence is the production of a repertoire of risks through which families confront as well as manage their reproductive behaviour. In this process, the full complexity and significance of any family's reproductive history can be lost, as they attempt to structure genetic information in a meaningful way. Experts' mobilising of the above concepts makes families' gathering of genetic information a complicated process, protracted over time.

One expert discussed a particular couple who perceived themselves at risk of an inherited genetic disorder. It was only after two pregnancies that their carrier status and genetic risk became clinical knowledge—knowledge which obviously affected their future reproductive choices. But, gaining definite knowledge involved the expert and family in building a picture of this particular couple's risk status. This was an erratic process, extending over three pregnancies.

> We had a couple . . . The mother's cousin has a child with (genetic
> disease) and they wanted a gene test . . . She was found to be a carrier. . . .
> During pregnancy, [she had] a spontaneous abortion and they forgot
> about it. . . . When we got the result, we . . . asked after the father's
> sample . . . It had not been taken. . . . We got the . . . sample . . . He was
> found to be a carrier too. So there was a risk in that family. They had a
> healthy child earlier. [After these pregnancies] they had another . . . which
> was an affected fetus . . . That was terminated also (A16 clinical geneticist)

One medical geneticist claimed that families wanted a sense of certainty about their risk status. He contended that for families to discover their level of risk was for them experienced as 'a relief'. In this context, Richards (1997) argues that the need for certainty about risk status is part of a general mentality in families, a mentality founded on a 'lay knowledge of inheritance'. Within this lay knowledge, families find relief in experts' assessments of their risk status. However, one expert claimed that assessing risk status may satisfy a family's need for certainty (*i.e.* 'to be sure') *regardless* of the result of their risk assessment (*i.e.* whether it is high or low):

> It is a relief for the family if they know that they can have a prenatal test . . . if you tell them that you have a Downs child but . . . you are young . . . and have a very small chance of having another. They ask, 'How high is our risk?' Let's say that it's one per cent . . . There is another family with a recessive disease with a high risk of 25 per cent. My experience is that where a family already has an abnormal child—whether it is a one per cent or 25 per cent [risk] does [not] make too much difference. They want to be sure about their next child. This is . . . the mentality of the families. They want to be sure [and it] does not make too much difference if it is one per cent or five per cent or 25 per cent. This is my experience (B5 medical geneticist).

One expert noted that side by side with a family's quest for certainty is the notion that information on their 'gene level' is more often than not uncertain. As families attempt to structure meaningful genetic information, they depend on expert certainty. The irony is that experts may not 'really know':

> There has been this huge development in genetics, so that we have been able to screen all possible things. . . . Of course the information is much more accurate, exact and certain. But still . . . you don't really know if you look at your family what you are going to expect. . . . even if you have the information on the gene level. There are very few diseases about which you really know what is going to happen (A15 lawyer).

Regardless of the perceived tension between uncertainty and certainty, some experts believe that most if not all families are 'eager' to find out their genetic makeup. Finding their genetic makeup was viewed as an opportunity 'to get to know what was possible' for them as a family. Therefore, 'knowing their genetic makeup' was perceived as having a certain status in the repertoire of families' reproductive choices. Experts claimed that at the very least knowing enabled families to identify the disease in their families and who it affects. Thus, a clinical geneticist said:

> They want to know what it means to the person who is affected, what sort of treatment can be offered and what are the causes of the disease. . . . [They want to know] anyone in the family who it concerns. So it can be . . . a young couple with a child who has . . . a genetic disorder and they want to know what all this means . . . If it is their first child, [they] want to

know whether this will affect subsequent children . . . and what the risks
are. . . . So I find myself in a sort of balancing [act] . . . in what I say to
people . . . (A17).

This 'balancing act' was all about assessing how much genetic knowledge
experts needed to provide if families wanted to be more certain of their possibilities 'as a family'. She continues:

Families . . . are eager to find out what is possible . . . I know a family
who had one son with a . . . severe genetic disorder and [he] died—the first
child . . . They are expecting a baby and they [want to] make sure that the
boy who died had this disorder . . . They are now expecting a girl. So . . .
though the boy had this disorder . . . the girl will not be at risk. And the
situation with this test is that the gene has been found . . . But not all have
been identified and sequenced . . . Part of the gene can be ripped out for
screening for mutations. If this can be done for this family, this will be a
useful result. If they find a mutation in one of the known parts of the
gene, the family will know (A17).

In a related context, a gynaecologist claimed that for some families,
knowing their genetic makeup could mean that they would not 'take that
risk again' (*i.e.* have an affected child):

Usually if the family . . . knows what it is to have a disabled child . . .
families do not want to take that risk again (A9).

The above comment suggests that some experts perceive families' need to
know their genetic make up as somehow empowering, if knowledge of risk
enables clearer reproductive choices. 'Knowing their genetic makeup'
implies that families have the resources to make important reproductive
choices which they, the experts, would help to facilitate. One expert asked
simply:

How do we actually use [our] knowledge in terms of empowering people
(D7)?

At the same time, experts' perceptions of 'families' need to know' tended
to lend support to cultural idioms, if not misconceptions: 'true' kinship is
genetic and a proper family is a domestic unit grounded in blood ties (Shore
1992: 300), or a 'proper' family is linked by a blood tie which, in turn, is
equated with a genetic tie (Strathern 1997: 48).

Experts claim that if a family is unable to fulfill 'true kinship' because of
what is identified as 'bad' genes, the family relies on an expert to ameliorate
its situation both now and in the future. In this alleviation process, some
experts may gain professional credibility, if not divine status (Rothman

1998b: 502). Yet, when experts detect 'bad genes', something 'wrong' or a defective 'child', this has wide implications, going beyond the clinical relationship. Simply, experts implicate most, if not all kinship ties, as one policy maker noted:

> It can be a great misery for the family and ruin their entire lives to bring into the world a child which has a . . . big defect . . . it is something very important in one's life to get a child with a big defect. . . . The lives not only of the child, the family and the parents but of all the family and the other children are affected by a child which is defective (B1).

If the key to reproduction is how 'good' genes mix, what people do to mix genes appears less important. Nonetheless, 'good' family planning emerges as a visible disciplinary practice which has been linked by families and experts to genetic assessment. For example, prenatal genetic testing has the potential to become a need (Beaulieu and Lippman 1995) as well as a lifestyle (Lippman 1994b) in our consumerist culture. Pregnant women and indeed 'pregnant couples' (Shildrick 1997: 23) tend to accept prenatal screening along with routine prenatal care (Press and Browner 1997), as genetic technologies become daily practice. Yet, some pregnant women, couples and families refuse prenatal genetic testing.

More significantly, an already captive, yet 'voluntary' population of families exists under the rubric of older non-controversial medical practices (*i.e.* family planning, planned parenthood and contraception services). One expert argued that it is through these traditional routes that the need for prenatal genetic testing becomes visible:

> In the hospitals there are services that give information on family planning . . . Within this . . ., a small part is prenatal screening . . . The idea of family planning [goes back] many years and they . . . are giving [genetic] information and counselling (B4 lawyer).

Another lawyer noted how involvement in family planning may lead to asking 'existential' questions, challenging families to consider newer technologies in traditional medical settings:

> In family planning we . . . inform [people] that it (*i.e.* prenatal genetic testing) is voluntary. We inform them . . . about the results or possible results. If you go on this program, [we ask] 'What does it mean for you, your children and the rest of your family' (A15)?

Linking reproductive genetics with older non-controversial medical practices, such as family planning, serves to fuse the interests of experts, families and the health care system—a strategy necessary for legitimation of further developments. Qureshi and Raeburn (1993) argue that people's contact with genetics, opportunistic or otherwise, facilitates their openness to it both in the short and long term. Placing genetic technologies within the domain of older non-controversial practices may encourage family compliance.

In this context, Jonsen (1996) contends that while the gathering of genomic information in a multiplicity of catchment sites will inevitably change the psychology of ordinary family life, it could be argued further that this information is needed equally by 'normal patient families' and experts alike (1996: 9). Maximising choice and genetic survival for an expert's 'patient family' may be one way of maximising beneficence for oneself (Lilford *et al*. 1994) as a valued expert and successful genetic story teller.

In the above discussions, I have explored the notion of experts as 'genetic story tellers' and producers of genetic ideology, and have examined the types of claims they construct as well as the impact of these claims. In the next part of the chapter, I offer a theoretical elaboration of experts' cultural production of genetics work and examine how in making their claims, experts employ a series of normative strategies.

## Doing 'genetics work': the need for normative strategies

How experts theorise about their work in telling genetic stories is illuminating. Here, the focus is on how, in doing genetics work and making their claims, experts employ a series of normative strategies in order to be successful genetic story tellers. Regardless of whether or not they share a consensus, experts employ these strategies to construct a theoretical base from their wealth of genetics intelligence. These strategies define what is needed for effective genetic story telling and include: (1) claiming ownership of genetic knowledge and practices; (2) maintaining a distinction between the social and scientific; (3) deploying genetic foundationalism; and (4) advocating the application of bioethics. These strategies, shaped by the prism of heritability, ensure, at the very least, a common frame of reference. But, what do these entail?

### Claiming ownership of genetic knowledge

In an attempt to ensure that the science of genetics will persist, experts claim ownership of genetic knowledge and resultant practices, while speculating on the potential health benefits of genetics. One expert expressed his approach to prenatal genetic screening as a 'mass medical activity' for disease prevention. He believes that this 'activity' is the domain of clinical genetics which, he implies, is a distinct discipline within biomedicine:

> Screening is an opportunity for preventing a serious disease . . . Here we have a mass screening test . . . My approach [to prenatal genetic screening] is basically as a mass medical activity. . . . This is still very much a specialist area covered by the clinical genetics discipline (D6 researcher).

A clinical geneticist explores this view further. She felt very strongly that only specialists should interpret genetics test results:

> I think . . . susceptibility tests in the hands of a geneticist or clinical geneticist are OK but when it spreads out to the whole medical profession, it is not OK. We recommend that all these patients come to the clinical genetics department . . . Doctors must know what they are doing when they interpret these tests (A4).

While the human genome may open up broad panoramas of information, ownership is about maintaining the boundaries of genetics—holding genes as medical property to be marketed and bargained over. Kimbrell (1993) says that genes are public material neatly shelved by their proprietors (*i.e.* experts) in the human body shop. While the course of a genetic disease does not change within these boundaries, the public is given the illusion that a particular diseased gene can change if it undergoes 'therapy'. Paradoxically, one clinical geneticist made it very clear that gene therapy has no 'practical meaning yet' and that the public often misunderstands it's current use:

> If we think about knowledge on medical aspects of genetics, I think there are many misconceptions. People often think that gene therapy is . . . being done and it is a very good thing . . . They have no idea that it is something that is only being tested in some labs. . . . It has no practical meaning yet (A5).

Still, genetic disease can only be expected, watched or wondered about by both patient and expert. Thus, as Jonsen (1996: 11) contends, the expert quest for understanding genetic diseases, and owning the problem, focuses attention on a shift from a practical to a theoretical, speculative science—from Scientia Activa to Scientia Contemplativa. Jonsen suggests that within reproductive genetics, the expert is compelled to look beyond the presenting patient: the expert is forced to theorise—to consider the relationships, experiences and emotions of the many, linked at the molecular level—both now and in the future. Thus, in order to be successful, experts need ownership, claiming as a continuous strategy, affecting both current ideas on their patients' pedigrees and any molecular eventualities.

*Maintaining a distinction between the social and scientific*
Biomedical experts, similar to other scientists (Latour and Woolgar 1986: 21), distinguish between the 'social' (*i.e.* behavioural processes) and the 'intellectual' (*i.e.* objective science). In their mind's eye, society is constructed as separate from the realm of science. In genetics, this issue has been flagged up by Anne Kerr and her colleagues. (See Kerr *et al.* 1997: 295). The reason for this distinction is that some experts may be threatened by the encroachment of external, social factors, particularly politics.

Regardless of the fact that some experts are keen to get 'politically' involved to advance the genetics cause, they view their biomedical activities as being driven by science not politics. While the distinction between the social and the scientific tends to be accepted as unproblematic, it may have significant consequences for the type of genetics experts produce. For example, experts' interests in the new genetics are spurred on by their scientific or intellectual interests—concerns that are constantly objectified. As the unchanging course of a disease unfolds, these concerns are 'followed' and 'described'. One expert illustrates this point quite vividly:

> As a geneticist, I have been very much interested in population genetics, learning how to approach populations *intellectually*. So I collected all the patients. . . . in the country . . . to follow their story and describe the natural history of the disease . . . (D4) (author's emphasis).

Elucidating this distinction further, another expert discussed what he saw as 'an intrusion from society' by politicians in his area of work. He believed they caused 'political problems' and thwarted his scientific role with their misplaced social interests. This obstetrician stated:

> What strikes me . . . is . . . the involvement of politicians and the ethical problems they see. . . . They have problems with screening, because . . . the end result . . . if something is found, . . . is an abortion. That's their problem. That's why they don't want to talk about it or when they talk about it, they only do it in negative terms . . . They always say, 'Oh it's no good because it will cost you a lot of abortions and there will be no advantages because handicapped people are no longer accepted in society'. . . . They only see the problems. . . . So the first thing I see in screening is . . . the political problems (C6).

This expert wanted to maintain a clear distinction between his scientific 'genetics' work and the 'social' (*e.g.* abortions and an interest in disability), perceived as disruptive to this work. In his comment, the 'social' values of politicians do not appear to sit well next to the 'intellectual' ones of the scientist. He wanted to make this mis-match clear. This is an example of how experts are able to draw upon this distinction between the 'social' and the 'scientific' as a powerful resource to characterise their own work. To be successful, they utilise this distinction to demonstrate the significance of themselves over and above others and more importantly, the intellectual (*i.e.* thoughtful, contemplative) nature of their work. This strategy is an elementary part of the experts' repertoire and is consistent with their use of 'gene talk' which, Conrad (1997) argues, functions to over-simplify very complex, social issues. As a strategy to maintain professional dominance vis a vis others outside the circle of science, they attempt to ensure the dominance of the intellectual by constantly opposing 'social' intrusions.

*The deployment of genetic foundationalism*

As part of the above-mentioned maintenance work, experts employ a type of genetics foundationalism upon which they are able to ground their scientific endeavours and, more importantly, exploit the cultural significance of their genetics work. McCaughey contends that 'foundationalism assumes the need for, and existence of, one authoritative framework for distinguishing the right from the wrong, the real from the unreal, and the healthy from the sick' (1993: 235). She argues that it is precisely this universalising tendency that reproduces 'the ability of those who already have privilege access to knowledge production to determine the normative framework and the inability of those with less access to knowledge production to challenge that framework with any credibility' (1993: 236). In this context, eugenics, the concern with the genetic improvement of mankind, becomes fundamental to genetics foundationalism (see Paul 1992: 667).

In discussing eugenics, one lawyer believed that a measure of whether or not genetics is eugenicist is how far it can go. Simply, 'how "preventative" (*i.e.* of disabilities) is it?' In her view, the more preventative, the more it was eugenicist:

> The more instruments you have in your hands to prevent disability, the less you come to accept it. It's [disability] something that can be avoided. It's preventive medicine but you don't know how far it will go. . . . You do all of this testing to prevent disabled babies being born with defects. . . . Will this turn to eugenics or not in the long run? . . . How far can preventive health go? Prevention [in] the extreme can become a sort of eugenics if you're preventing things more and more (B7).

In contrast, a clinical geneticist claimed that as a word, eugenics, has a bad press and that she wanted to emphasise its 'good side':

> If we take the word, eugenics . . . people . . . think of the worst things— . . . the evil, bad things that you can do with genetics. Well it is not [like that]. Eugenics was a good word at that time when it was used for the whole field of human genetics. We wanted then to improve the . . . quality of the human race. This side of the word has to be considered more. When we offer these tests, our intentions are to improve the quality of the human race . . . (A4).

Another defender of eugenics said simply:

> My view is that the principle of abortion for disabling handicaps for serious disorders that cause disability is acceptable, however, disagreeable that may be (D6 researcher).

In a foundationalist framework, experts express eugenicist concerns. In this way, they attempt to facilitate successful genetic story telling as well as the productive circulation of a genetics moral order in which one's genetic capital (*i.e.* genes) becomes a reproductive resource within the family (Ettorre forthcoming). Simply, they want to privilege a morality of the body which upholds the standard for conventional (*i.e.* non-diseased, genetically 'normal') offspring and society's need for citizens who are fit to be born.

*Advocating the application of bioethics*
While experts may employ genetics foundationalism as a way of making politics and other extraneous social factors unimportant, if not invisible, in their knowledge production process, they need continually to ensure that *all* relevant normative issues are incorporated into the domain of the intellectual. Indeed, they do this by advocating the application of bioethics which functions to maintain the significance of the intellectual (*i.e.* autonomy of science), while, at the same time, staking a claim in the social (*i.e.* morality). In practice, this means that if ethical problems arise these can be identified by experts within the context of science, and transmitted to the public as accessible, 'social' rather than 'scientific' knowledge. For example, while the medical model of pregnancy may be both 'product orientated' and 'fetocentric' (Rothman 1996: 26), the strategies employed by those upholding this model are utilised to ensure optimum reproductive health outcomes within society (Bobinski 1996: 80). This model and its attendant strategies are justified on ethical grounds because health and life are valued over disease and death. In these contexts, reproductive genetics can be seen to rest on firm ethical grounds. As Rothman says:

> Ethicists who evaluate prenatal diagnosis are often most comfortable with those situations in which the fetus is diagnosed with an inevitably fatal condition: it might not survive the pregnancy, or even if brought to term and born alive would die shortly thereafter. In such circumstances, prenatal diagnosis is generally understood to present no-ethical dilemma. An abortion simply brings the inevitable to a rapid conclusion (1996: 26).

In considering prenatal diagnosis, one ethicist believes that as decisions about abortions become more public so also will 'the moral question' (*i.e.* ethics of selective abortion). In her view, this will have far-reaching social implications:

> The really important issue is what is going to be done after you hear about the results. This is a moral question and I think this is a question of motherhood and [for] each one of us (B9).

Nevertheless, to be successful, experts need to ensure that genetics work is done in spite of moral or ethical implications. While experts can be seen to embody paternalism, their authority is deemed worthy of respect and may be appealing for patient and expert alike. The information experts produce may be difficult to refuse or resist. One expert, both a lawyer and ethicist, discussed how easy it could be for some women to be drawn into an expert's mindset, even though they are 'given the choice' to refuse testing:

> You know doctors are more paternalistic . . . They have a . . . traditional role . . . Their authority may be more respected than in other areas. . . . Women are given the choice. For example, you can . . . or if you don't want, you don't [have to] take the tests. But they are given the information in such a way that it is difficult for them to refuse (B7).

Here, in order to be sustained as a viable scientific discourse, reproductive genetics is aided by the moral mediation of experts. Without this, there is a danger that part of the genetics order will break down and expert story telling will become unsuccessful. Nevertheless, while ethics is a fundamental piece of the knowledge base of genetics and helps to produce this genetics order, ethics is constructed in a piecemeal way. Simply, most if not all experts agree on the need for ethics and are keenly aware of the ethical dimensions of their work. However, their views on the scope, importance and function of ethics tends to vary. Some believe ethics is fundamental in their work; others believe ethics, while important, is relative and still others question whether or not experts could 'hold a view' on ethics (Ettorre 1996).

Yet, experts are expected to 'practice', if not embody, ethics. Thus, telling genetic stories may mean providing ethical codes for genetic material. Experts fashion powerful judgements about genes, ethics and indeed health through relatively stable ensembles of procedures, instruments, theories, results, and products to which they give their allegiance (Wright 1994: 13). In turn, their judgements filter through society and help to construct the view that all adverse consequences of social, psychological, economic and physical functioning flow not only from illness but also from genes (Asch and Geller 1996). More significantly, expert judgements can become the engine for further developments in genetics, as ethics and technological advances become inextricably linked.

In this context, one expert suggested that the concern for ethics should go hand in hand with the growth of technology. In a very curious way, his statement was a defence of technological development, privileged over ethics. But, for him it was difficult to consider the 'rights' and 'wrongs' of an issue, when new technologies were being developed at such a fast pace.

This policy maker said:

> When science and new technologies develop [it] is sexy, . . . attractive, interesting and exciting. Everybody wants to push back the barriers . . . instead of saying every now and then, 'Should we be pausing and saying, "Is this something we ought to do? [and] not, "Is this something we can do?" The time to say that it is something we ought to do is five years before we can do it . . . That's when you need to, before it's in place. Once

it's in place, it is very difficult to say, 'No, we ought not to be doing this'.
. . . You need to do it in advance . . . The problem is that when the
scientists say immediately 'It's available now', it is very difficult to resist it
being used . . . We have to start saying, 'Now we have limited ability to
do . . . genetic testing'. But it's going to escalate very rapidly. We need to
be making the decisions now about where we put pegs in the sand and
where we decide what is right and wrong (D7).

This excerpt illustrates the type of inner logic of science or 'reflexive scienti-
zation', highlighted by Beck (1992: 159–60) in his observations on science in
the risk society. The portal through which genetic risk is opened up and
treated scientifically is a critique of science and its attendant technologies.
Based on social definitions and relations, these risks destroy opportunities
to resolve mistakes internally (i.e. within science). Scientific expansion and
development presuppose self-criticism. Attempts by experts to resolve technological mistakes are transmitted publicly—achieving moral significance.
While these publicly transmitted judgements become forced critiques of new
developments, a complex legitimating process occurs, creating further technological expansion.

Ethics may appear to function in this context as a check on technology.
But, ethics can also be employed strategically as an intellectual bulldozer
pressing the frontiers of science. As Rothman (1998a: 36) aptly states,
'bioethics becomes a translator, sometimes an apologist, sometimes an
enabler of scientific "progress" '. Experts hope to eliminate genetic abnormalities in offspring. They do this either by biological prevention or apparent genetic cure (i.e. gene therapy). In this quest for healthy babies, experts
may experience a moral imperative to push the boundaries of science further
(Spallone 1995: 129). Ethics allows them to be prosperous and to do just
that.

### Conclusion: the need for sociological vigilance

The contention in this chapter has been that as 'genetic story tellers', experts
produce ways of thinking or ideologies, shaped by the prism of genetics and
notions of risk and cultural constructions of patient families and kinship
ties. While knowledge of genetic makeup within families is perceived as
empowering by some experts, this knowledge is constructed as a need which
becomes routinised within older, more established health care settings. In
short, risk knowledge within families translates into reproductive choices,
interpreted and mediated by experts.

To be successful story tellers, experts attempt to ensure the 'correct' theoretical pathways for the development of their scientific interests as well as
the science of genetics itself. This is done by employing a series of normative

strategies. In a cultural arena, marked by the social construction of biological phenomena, they mobilise knowledge and practice ownership, the split between society and science, genetic foundationalism and bioethics as strategic devices under the banner of genetics. Their knowledge claims and attempts at knowledge building reflect their interests concerning the role of genetics in reproduction.

While this chapter reports on findings from an empirical study on European experts, and offers a theoretical elaboration on experts' use of normative strategies in reproductive genetics, the issues it raises can be framed by the sociology of knowledge. In this context, as genetic experts articulate, construct and reproduce their positions of authority they fulfill important social and scientific roles as interpreters of knowledge. These experts represent specialists: reproductive invigilators, fulfilling the cultural need in the population for genetic supervision and 'know how'. In this invigilation process, they embody educators, surveillors and story tellers whose role it is to reinforce and legitimate a genetic order, required for the common good.

As sociologists, we have the important task of uncovering some of the unintended consequences of the new genetics. At the same time, we must recognise that the issues are enormously difficult and socially complex. We must be vigilant because, as Haraway (1990) argues, the intellectual issues that these experts are concerned with are deeply intertwined with social and political questions concerning the privileging of scientific knowledge and nature over ethical values and social issues. Reproductive genetics embodies complex social relationships and experts involved in these relationships are key players in cultures where genetic knowledge is being valued increasingly on a daily basis.

## Acknowledgements

This work is part of research programme 'The development of prenatal screening in Europe: the past, the present and the future', funded by the European Commission (BIOMED II—Contract No. BMH4–CT96–0740) and includes research partners from the Department of Sociology, University of Helsinki, Finland; the Health Service Research Unit of the National Research and Development Centre for Welfare and Health, Helsinki, Finland; the Department of Epidemiology and Health Promotion, National Public Health Institute, Helsinki, Finland; the Department of Preschool Education, University of Athens, Greece; the Institute of Child Health, Athens, Greece; the Northern Centre for Health Care Research, University of Groningen, The Netherlands; the Social Science Research Unit, University of London, UK. I should like to thank: my research partners for their help in carrying out this research, all of the experts who participated in this study and who remain anonymous, the editors and the reviewers for their valuable comments on earlier drafts of this chapter.

## Note

1   In order to maintain the anonymity of respondents, interviews are coded by the letters A, B, C and D followed by relevant interview numbers.

## References

Asch, A. and Geller, G. (1996) Feminism, bioethics and genetics. In Wolfe, S. (ed) *Feminism and Bioethics: Beyond Reproduction*. New York: Oxford University Press.

Asch, D.A., Hershey, J.C., Pauly, M.V., Patton, J.P., Jedrziewski, M.K. and Mennuti, M.T. (1996) Genetic screening for reproductive planning: methodological and conceptual issues in policy analysis, *American Journal of Public Health*, 86, 5, 684–90.

Beaulieu, A. and Lippman, A. (1995) 'Everything you need to know': how women's magazines structure prenatal diagnosis for women over 35, *Women and Health*, 23, 3, 59–74.

Beck, U. (1992) *The Risk Society: Towards a New Modernity*. London: Sage.

Beekhuis, J.R. (1993) *Maternal Serum Screening for Fetal Down's Syndrome and Neural Tube Defects: a Prospective Study, Performed in the North of the Netherlands*. Groningen: National University.

Bobinski, M.A. (1996) Genetics and reproductive decision making. In Murray, T., Rothstein, M.A. and Murray, R.F. (eds) *The Human Genome Project and the Future of Health Care*. Bloomington: Indiana University Press.

Brock, D.J.H., Kent, P., Morris, J., Doherty, R.A., Bradley, L.A., Haddow, J.E., Toegerson, D.J., Walters, S., Cuckle, H.S., Richardson, G.A. and Sheldon, T.A. (1996) Cost effectiveness of antenatal screening for cystic fibrosis, *British Medical Journal*, 312, 7035, 908–10.

Calnan, M. (1987) *Health and Illness: the Lay Perspective*. London: Tavistock.

Clarke, A. (1997) Introduction. In Clarke, A. and Parsons, E. (ed) *Culture, Kinship and Genes: towards Cross-Cultural Genetics*. Houndsmills: Macmillan.

Conrad, P. (1997) Public eyes and private genes: historical frames, news constructions and social problems, *Social Problems*, 44, 2, 139–54.

Cowan, R.S. (1994) Women's roles in the history of amniocentesis and chorionic villi sampling. In Rothenberg, K. and Thomson, E.J. (eds) *Women and Prenatal Testing: Facing the Challenges of Genetic Testing*. Columbus, Ohio: Ohio State University Press.

Davison, C., Davey Smith, G. and Frankel, S. (1991) Lay epidemiology and the prevention paradox: the implications of coronary candidacy for health education, *Sociology of Health and Illness*, 13, 1–19.

Duster, T. (1990) *Backdoor to Eugenics*. New York: Routledge.

Ettorre, E. (1996) *The New Genetics Discourse in Finland: Exploring Experts' Views within Surveillance Medicine*. Helsinki: Suomen Kuntaliitto (Association of Finnish Metropolitan Authorities).

Ettorre, E. (1997) The complexities of genetic technologies: unintended consequences and responsible ethics, *Sosiaalilääketieteelinen Aikakauslehti (Journal of Finnish Social Medicine)*, 34, 257–67.

Ettorre, E. (forthcoming) *Reproductive Genetics, Gender and the Body*. London and New York: Routledge.

Ettorre, E., Adams, E., Alderson, P., Aro, A., Dragonas, T., Hemminki, E., Tymstra, T. and Van de Hueval, W. (1997) *Annual Activity Report of the European Union Project on the Development of Prenatal Screening in Europe: the Past, the Present and the Future*. Helsinki: University of Helsinki.

Ettorre, E., Adams, E., Alderson, P., Aro, A., Dragonas, T., Hemminki, E., Tymstra, T. and Van de Hueval, W. (1999) *Final Report of the European Union Project on the Development of Prenatal Screening in Europe: the Past, the Present and the Future*. Helsinki: University of Helsinki.

Faden, R. (1994) Reproductive genetic testing, prevention and the ethics of mothering. In Rothenberg, K. and Thomson, E.J. (eds) *Women and Prenatal Testing: Facing the Challenges of Genetic Testing*. Columbus, Ohio: Ohio State University Press.

Giddens, A. (1991) *The Consequences of Modernity*. Cambridge: Polity Press.

Haraway, D. (1990) A manifesto for Cyborgs: science, technology and socialist feminism in the 1980s. In Nicholson, L.J. (ed) *Feminism/Postmodernism*. London and New York: Routledge.

Heinonen, S., Ryynänen, M., Kirkinen, P., Penttilä, I., Syrjänen, K., Seppala, M. and Saarikoski, S. (1996) Prenatal screening for congenital nephrosis in East Finland: results and impact on the birth prevalence of the disease, *Prenatal Diagnosis*, 16, 207–13.

Higgs, P. (1997) The limits of medical knowledge. In Scambler, G. (ed) *Sociology as Applied to Medicine*. London: W.B. Saunders.

Jonsen, A.R. (1996) The impact of mapping the human genome on the patient–physician relationship. In Murray, T., Rothstein, M.A. and Murray, R.F. (eds) *The Human Genome Project and the Future of Health Care*. Bloomington: Indiana University Press.

Kerr, A., Cunningham-Burley, S. and Amos, A. (1997) The new genetics: professionals' discursive boundaries, *Sociological Review*, 45, 2, 297–303.

Kimbrell, A. (1993) *The Human Body Shop*. San Francisco: Harper.

Latour, B. and Woolgar, S. (1986) *Laboratory Life: the Construction of Scientific Facts*. Princeton, New Jersey: Princeton University Press (2nd Edition).

Lilford, R.J., Vanderkerckhove, P. and Thornton, J.G. (1994) Decision analysis in clinical genetics, *Bailliere's Clinical Obstetrics and Gynaecology*, 8, 3, 625–42.

Lippman, A. (1992) Led (astray) by genetic maps: the cartography of the human genome and health care, *Social Science and Medicine*, 35, 12, 1469–76.

Lippman, A. (1994a) Prenatal genetic testing and screening: constructing needs and reinforcing inequities. In Clark, A. (ed) *Genetic Counselling: Practice and Principles*. London: Routledge.

Lippman, A. (1994b) The genetic construction of prenatal testing. In Rothenberg, K. and Thompson, E.J. (eds) *Women and Prenatal Testing: Facing the Challenges of Genetic Testing*. Columbus, Ohio: Ohio State University Press.

Mahowald, M.B. (1994) Reproductive genetics and gender justice. In Rothenberg, K. and Thomson, E.J. (eds) *Women and Prenatal Testing: Facing the Challenges of Genetic Testing*. Columbus, Ohio: Ohio State University Press.

Mantingh, A., Breed, A.J.P.M., Bukhuis, J.R. and van Lith, J.M.M. (1991) *Screening in Prenatal Diagnosis*. (Proceedings of an international symposium on screening in prenatal diagnosis). Groningen: Academic Press.

Marteau, T.M. (1995) Towards informed decisions about prenatal testing: a review, *Prenatal Diagnosis*, 15, 1215–26.

McCaughey, M. (1993) Evolution, ethics and the search for uncertainty, *Science as Culture*, 4, 2, 212–43.

Parsons, E. and Atkinson, P. (1993) Genetic risk and reproduction, *Sociological Review*, 679–706.

Paul, D.B. (1992) Eugenic anxieties, social realities and political choices, *Social Research*, 59, 3, 663–83.

Press, N. and Browner, C.H. (1997) Why women say yes to prenatal diagnosis, *Social Science and Medicine*, 45, 7, 979–89.

Qureshi, N. and Raeburn, J.A. (1993) Clinical genetics meets primary care, *British Medical Journal*, 307, 816–17.

Richards, M.P.M. (1993) The new genetics: some issues for social scientists, *Sociology of Health and Illness*, 15, 5, 567–86.

Richards, M. (1997) It runs in the family: lay knowledge about inheritance. In Clarke, A. and Parsons, E. (eds) *Culture, Kinship and Genes: Towards Cross-Cultural Genetics*. Houndsmills: Macmillan.

Rosner, M. and Johnson, T.R. (1995) Telling stories: metaphors of the Human Genome Project, *Hypatia*, 10, 4, 104–29.

Rothenberg, K. (1996) Feminism, law and ethics, *Kennedy Institute of Ethics Journal*, 6, 1, 69–84.

Rothman, B.K. (1994) *The Tentative Pregnancy: Amniocentesis and the Sexual Politics of Motherhood*. London: Pandora.

Rothman, B.K. (1996) Medical sociology confronts the human genome, *Medical Sociology News*, December, 22, 1, 23–35.

Rothman, B.K. (1998a) *Genetic Maps and Human Imaginations*. New York: W.W. Norton.

Rothman, B.K. (1998b) A sociological sceptic in the brave new world, *Gender and Society*, 12, 3, 501–4.

Shildrick, M. (1997) *Leaky Bodies and Boundaries: Feminism, Postmodernism and (Bio)ethics*. London–New York: Routledge.

Shore, C. (1992) Virgin births and sterile debates, *Current Anthropology*, 33, 3, 295–314.

Spallone, P. (1995) Bad conscience and collective unconscious: science, discourse and reproductive technology. In Rosenback, B. and Schott, R.M. (eds) *For Plantning, Kon og Teknologi*. Copenhagen: Museum Tusculanums Forlag.

Steinberg, D.L. (1997) *Bodies in Glass: Genetics, Eugenics, Embryo Ethics*. Manchester and New York: Manchester University Press.

Strathern, M. (1997) The work of culture: an anthropological perspective. In Clarke, A. and Parsons, E. (eds) *Culture, Kinship and Genes: Towards Cross-Cultural Genetics*. Houndsmills: Macmillan.

Tymstra, Tjeerd (1991) Prenatal diagnosis, prenatal screening and the rise of the tentative pregnancy, *International Journal of Technology Assessment*, 7, 4, 509–16.

Wald, N., Brock, D., Haddow, J. and Doherty, R.A. (1995) Antenatal screening for cystic fibrosis, *British Medical Journal*, 310, 6988, 1199.

Wald, N.J., Densem, J.W., George, L., Muttukrishna, S. and Knight, P.G. (1996) Prenatal screening for Downs's syndrome using Inhibin-A as a serum marker, *Prenatal diagnosis*, 16, 143–53.

Wendell, Susan (1992) Toward a feminist theory of disability. In Holmes, H.B. and Purdy, L. (eds) *Feminist Perspectives in Medical Ethics*. Bloomington: Indiana University Press.

Wright, S. (1994) *Molecular Politics: Developing American and British Regulatory Policy for Genetic Engineering*, 1972–82. Chicago: University of Chicago Press.

# The human drama of genetics: 'hard' and 'soft' media representations of inherited breast cancer

## Lesley Henderson and Jenny Kitzinger

### Introduction

The media are a crucial source of public information about health and illness (Chapman and Lupton 1994, Miller *et al.* 1998, Philo 1999). However, the conflicting priorities of scientific and media communities have been well documented (Friedman *et al.* 1986, Karpf 1988, Wilkie 1991, Nelkin 1996, Peters 1995). Certainly, the media do not necessarily prioritise the risks judged to be most important by epidemiologists, doctors or scientists. Media values are not the same as those of 'the experts' (Kitzinger 1999).

One approach to examining the coverage of scientific issues is to track the media reporting of articles from key journals, such as *Nature* or the *British Medical Journal* (*BMJ*). Such studies tend to focus on news around scientific discoveries (Miller 1995) or specialist reports on the science and health pages (Entwhistle 1995, Moyer *et al.* 1995). However, there is also widespread acknowledgement that broader representations of science (such as those expressed through the Frankenstein metaphor) may also be crucial (Turney 1998) and that 'the gene' has become a cultural icon in the broadest sense (Nelkin and Lindee 1995). Studies of public understandings of biomedicine have highlighted how images from popular fiction may be referenced in public discourse (Kerr *et al.* 1998) and have pointed to the role of non-news outlets such as women's magazines (Richards *et al.* 1995). A recent Wellcome Trust study of 'Public perspectives on human cloning' concludes that research participants' concerns about the social implications of this science 'were often described in the context of popular cultural imagery such as science fiction films and media stories portraying the lives of public figures. Scientific news coverage appeared to have a lesser impact upon views' (The Wellcome Trust 1998: 4).

In studying how breast cancer genetics was reported in the media we could have focused solely on the reporting surrounding the discoveries of the two 'breast cancer genes': BRCA1 and BRCA2 (reported in 1994 and 1995 respectively). However, to examine such reporting in isolation would have ignored the way in which these discoveries diffused into the media and became integrated into a 'cultural repertoire' for understanding inherited risk. This chapter reports our work into media reporting which adopted a broader approach, including exploring how inherited/genetic risk translated from the hard news arena into human interest stories, women's magazines 'true life tales' and fiction. We use this study to argue for a three-dimensional approach to studying the media which takes into account the importance of human interest approaches to science coverage.

## Methods

This chapter draws on research, funded by the NHS Executive, designed to examine how media representations of breast cancer were shaped, what form the coverage took, and how this might influence public understandings. The project involved three intertwined levels of enquiry.

1 The first stage was an analysis of media production processes. This involved interviews with journalists (including medical/science specialists, feature writers and non specialists) and also with documentary makers, scriptwriters and magazine editors. We also interviewed press officers from cancer charities as well as relevant pressure groups, In total, 40 interviews were completed (mostly lasting half an hour to an hour). These were tape-recorded and transcribed. All interviews were conducted by Lesley Henderson.

2 The second stage of the research was an analysis of media content. This involved two main samples. We monitored a selection of press coverage for three years (1995–1997). We also collected a broader sample which included television, magazines and radio for a four-month period (September–December 1997).

3 The third stage of the research focused on audience reception of the coverage. This was explored through 30 tape-recorded focus group discussions which were then transcribed and coded onto the data analysis programme, NUDIST. Twenty-five groups were conducted with women with no known special interest in breast cancer. These women (from a range of backgrounds and areas in Britain) were accessed through community centres, clubs and work places. For example, the sample included people who worked together (*e.g.* waitresses) and groups who met for social, political or support purposes (*e.g.* a bridge club, a youth group, a black women's community group and members of an 'over 60s' group). The aim was to access a diverse range of women and to facilitate relaxed discussion. Where possible, sessions were conducted in places familiar to participants, such as their local community centre or, sometimes, in women's own homes. In addition to these 25 groups with 'ordinary women', a further five sessions were conducted with medical practitioners, breast cancer support workers and breast cancer survivors. In total there were 164 group participants (143 'ordinary women' and 21 people with special interest in the issue). The average group involved five or six participants and lasted between one and two hours. Most of the sessions were facilitated by Cherise Saywell (see Saywell *et al.* 1999).

The research was not designed to focus on genetics per se. However, this soon emerged as an important issue at every level. Inherited/genetic risk received a large proportion of media attention, it was frequently mentioned by journalists as a key story and it was raised spontaneously by participants in the focus groups. As we will demonstrate, however, both media reporting and public discussion often addressed the issue without framing it as a story about science. The focus was often more on family history or inheritance. The significance of this will become clear later, here we just wish to note that this is why we use the term 'inherited/genetic' risk.

## The media coverage: introducing the two samples

As this chapter focuses on media content we shall describe the methods for this part of the research in greater detail. The aim was (a) to look at a substantial amount of coverage over a long time scale and (b) to examine a range of coverage across different media outlets. To achieve this we had two sampling strategies. First, we examined three years of press coverage (1995–97) in eight different newspapers. The newspapers were selected to reflect different readership/political profiles.[1] We chose two daily 'tabloids' (newspapers with a large and predominantly working class readership): *The Sun* and *The Mirror*. We also examined three 'broadsheets', (newspapers with a narrower and predominantly middle class readership): *The Guardian*, *The Independent*, and *The Times*. In addition, we included three broadsheet Sunday newspapers (*The Observer*, *The Independent* and *The Sunday Times*). Articles were located from the tabloids via a manual search, but CD rom searches were used to identify articles in the broadsheets. The search terms used included words such as mammography and mastectomy in addition to breast cancer to ensure we accessed all relevant articles. Those which simply referenced breast cancer in passing (*e.g.* obituaries) were then excluded.

This three-year sampling strategy generated 708 news reports, feature articles, editorials and columns. These were coded onto a specially designed computer programme to allow for systematic quantitative analysis. Each item was indexed by headline, journalist's name and specialism, newspaper and page on which it appeared. We also recorded the main focus of each item (*e.g.* 'causes', 'screening' or 'treatment'). Additional details were coded such as the type of images used, which risk factors were mentioned, the use of statistics and which sources were cited.

This three-year sample of press reporting (N=708) was complemented by a second sample which covered a substantially shorter time period (September–December 1997) but which included a broader range of media. This included all national UK newspapers and the 10 top-selling women's magazines as well as television news, documentaries, chat shows, soaps and a selection of radio programmes. In addition, we monitored the *TV Times* during the course of the project (1997–1998) and recorded additional items where advance publicity indicated that they were about breast cancer.

In the next section we focus on our first sample: the three-year sample of press reporting. We use this to present some basic statistics about the profile of inherited/genetic risk in the newspapers and highlight the emphasis on human interest accounts. We then draw on our sampling from television, magazines and radio to illustrate how this emphasis ran through other media outlets too and to give a flavour of the nature of this reporting.

### Inherited risk: the media profile of 'family' breast cancer

*The quantity of coverage*
The first important finding from our content analysis is the high level of media attention devoted to inherited/genetic risk relative to other risks. This high profile was evident at several levels. Analysis of the eight selected newspapers for the three years identified 708 articles about breast cancer (excluding letters to the editor). One-hundred-and-fifty-two of these focused on risk factors for breast cancer and 51 focused on genetics/inheritance. In other words, genetics (or inherited risk) was the main topic of one out of every three articles focused on discussing risks.

In addition, family history was often mentioned *in passing* in articles about other aspects of breast cancer. In fact the only risk factor to be referenced more often was age.[2] Thus inherited/genetic risk had a much higher profile than a host of non-genetic factors which might modify the risks of breast cancer, including the contraceptive pill, HRT, pregnancy, hormones, class, diet or smoking (see Figure 1). This is in spite of the fact that BRCA1 and BRCA2 are believed to account for just five to 10 per cent of breast cancers (Easton *et al.* 1994, Wooster *et al.* 1994).

*The nature of the coverage and its diffusion into different formats and diverse media outlets*
The second important finding, evident from our content analysis, concerned *diffusion* of coverage. Analysis of our three-year sample showed that the issue of inherited/genetic risk had permeated beyond the traditional news format. Less than half of the reports about genetics/inheritance were news reports (n=21). The rest were features or personal accounts (n=25) or took other forms such as personal observations by columnists *e.g.* 'Why I won't search for the deadly gene' (Nigella Lawson *The Times* 28 February 1996). In addition, inherited risk was not just discussed on the science/health pages, but also appeared in readers' stories, on advice pages and even, in one instance, on the fashion page. *The Mirror* published a feature entitled: 'The secret fear I share with mum: TV's Leslie tells of her cancer scare' (17 May 1995). This showed television actor, Leslie Ash, modelling a 'short and snazzy: bright orange dress £520, by Moschino' and 'gold strappy evening shoes £49.99'. The article did include a brief discussion of Leslie Ash's feelings and fears about the 'hereditary disease' of breast cancer, but was primarily being used to promote clothing sales.

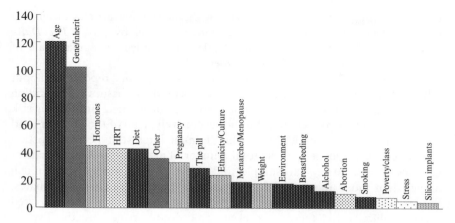

Figure 1   *Showing the number of articles referencing different potential risk factors for breast cancer**

• This is based on analysis of *all* references to any risk factor in the 708 articles about breast cancer which appeared in eight newspapers, 1995–97. Some articles concentrated entirely on one risk factor, others referenced more than one factor in passing, some made no mention of risk factors at all. The age of a woman was usually only mentioned as a risk factor in an implicit way. Press articles which contained statements such as 'she was only 33 so it was a shock to have cancer' were coded as referencing age as a risk factor.

Most of the reporting of inherited/genetic breast cancer, however, fell clearly into one of four categories: (a) scientific discoveries; (b) debates about testing; (c) controversies over patenting; (d) 'human interest stories'.

Early reporting focused on the first of these categories. The discoveries of BRCA1 and BRCA2 were reported on the front page and discussed within regular science/medical slots. The discovery of BRCA1 was announced prior to the start of our sample (in 1994). Even so, genetic discoveries (mainly around BRCA2) accounted for 18 per cent of the reports about genetics in our three-year sample. Headlines included: 'UK scientists claim breast cancer gene breakthrough' (*The Independent* 21 December 1995); 'Breast cancer gene isolated' (*The Guardian* 21 December 1995) and 'Second gene linked to breast cancer' (*The Times* 21 December 1995).

However, long after the announcement of the discoveries of BRCA1 and BRCA2, inherited/genetic risk continued to attract media interest in other ways. Controversy around insurance and patenting, for example, generated extensive debate, at least within the broadsheets, particularly in response to European directives. Discussion about patenting accounted for 26 per cent of the articles about breast cancer genetics in our sample *e.g.* 'Protest over patents goes global' (*The Times* 6 December 1995); 'Whose genes are they anyway?' (*Independent on Sunday* 9 November 1997). Similarly, a flurry of reports mentioning breast cancer followed the publication of a code of practice by the Advisory Committee on Genetic Testing. Debates about testing were the primary focus of 21 per cent of the newspaper articles discussing breast cancer genetics *e.g.* 'Alarm at genetic testing by post' (*The Daily Telegraph* 24 September 1997) and 'Codes of practice to regulate sale of DIY gene tests' (*The Times* 24 September 1997).

However, the single most dominant strand of reporting about inherited/genetic risk during 1995–1997 focused on issues surrounding prophylactic mastectomies and the experiences of women from 'high risk families'. This was particularly, but not exclusively, true of the popular (and more widely read) tabloid press. This 'human interest' type of reporting accounted for 27 per cent of the total number of articles about breast cancer genetics in our three-year sample and these articles were usually much longer than those about the gene discoveries, patenting or testing debates. Stories about individual women's feelings and dilemmas often covered several columns and there were even some double page spreads. Typical headlines included: 'Cutting deadly odds: These sisters are healthy yet they each want both breasts removed' (*The Mirror* 29 May 1996); 'Women at risk of cancer agonise over mastectomy' (*The Times* 26 February 1996); 'I didn't want to wait for it to come and get me' (*The Guardian* 29 April 1996) and 'Big sacrifice for survival' (*The Mirror* 6 May 1997).

These types of article are worth close examination as they formed a distinct genre of coverage which recycled similar narrative and images. A feature article in *The Observer* headlined 'The Breast Cancer Family' (*The Observer* 30 June 1996) condensed many of the main themes in its opening paragraph:

> Her mother died of it. Her aunt has it. She'll get it too. And her three daughters? 'I'm young and healthy and I'm going to have my breasts cut off. That sounds so ghastly. And of course I'm scared. What will I look like? What will I feel like? How will I cope and what will I become, who will I be?' (*The Observer* 30 June 1996)

Such stories were frequently accompanied by reproductions of women's wedding photographs or portraits showing them with their mothers or daughters. *The Mirror*, for example, reproduced three such images under the headline '9 of my family got breast cancer so I had my breasts removed in case I was the next' (*The Mirror* 14 February 1996). One picture showed the extended family with the subtitle 'A picture of tragedy', another displayed a diagram of 'Wendy's tragic family tree' representing those who carried 'the cancer gene' as black circles and squares.

It was these types of images and stories which were also reflected in a wide range of media over and above the newspapers. Stories based on 'high risk families' appeared in women's magazines, TV chat shows and documentaries. They also featured in soap operas and radio fiction. It is here that our broader sampling strategy which included magazines, television and radio provided useful additional data, especially as our focus group work showed that it was these types of stories and variety of outlets that had made most impression on women's understandings of genetic risk.

Accounts about breast cancer outside traditional news slots were often less about 'science' than about family relationships, drama and dilemmas. They frequently appeared in slots traditionally reserved for the exploration of sexuality and emotions. An article in the women's magazine, *Bella*, for example, explored the impact of the breast cancer gene on a woman and her partner. This was placed in a regular slot within the magazine called: 'Relationships: how we got through it' (*Bella* 8 October 1997). Two documentaries about genetic breast cancer also emphasised relationships and family dynamics. The BBC2's documentary *Homeground* (13 May 1997) told the same story as the *Bella* article, while Channel 4's *The Decision: Living in the Shadow* followed another woman, Wendy Watson, and her family through the genetic testing and decision-making process (27 February 1996). This latter episode was part of a series devoted to difficult medical dilemmas, and borrowed much from the detective genre as it portrayed Watson's quest to trace her family history and eventual discovery that nine relatives had contracted breast cancer at a young age. Narrative suspense was maintained by Wendy Watson's own test results too—a test which had only become available *after* she had undergone prophylactic surgery.

Inherited risk did not just feature in 'true stories' and documentaries, producers of fictional programmes also recognised the potential of such accounts. Women with a family history of breast cancer were the focus of two fictional representations during the course of our research project: a storyline in the medical soap opera, *Peak Practice* (ITV 12 January 1998) and a radio play (Radio 4 *The Monday Play* 19 May 1997). The former followed a young woman's discovery of a breast lump, her emotions around her own mother's early death, her desires for a double mastectomy and her fears for her daughter. The Radio 4 play echoed similar themes with its focus on 'Joy' and her sister 'Vita'. The plot of this drama also paralleled that of *The Decision* in following the two sisters through the process of being tested and discovering the results. Drama was heightened by the device of making Joy have 'the gene' while Vita does not. The play explored how genetic knowledge may ricochet through family relationships. Dramatic tensions were further increased by Joy's decision to become pregnant with eggs donated by her sister.

Both the radio play and the episode of *Peak Practice* explored the human cost of knowledge and explored uncertainty. Neither suggested that science and medicine offered clear-cut solutions. Indeed, in the radio play, as Joy considers prophylactic treatment, her husband asks: 'What is this? Self-destruction? Self-preservation?' She replies: 'Aren't they the same thing for me now?'. He responds by stating simply: 'What a mess.'

We have described these media representations in some detail to illustrate the saturation of certain themes and story lines across different media formats/outlets and to highlight the way in which this one aspect of risk became widely reported across a range of coverage using very similar motifs. Other dimensions of the story (such as scientific discoveries or patenting debates) did not have such broad attraction for the media.

This permeation of one aspect of the inherited/genetic risk issue has important implications for the *amount* of overall coverage for two reasons. First, if an issue is addressed in a range of different formats/outlets then the media's *'carrying capacity'* for that issue is greatly increased (Hilgartner and Bosk 1988). Secondly, such diffusion may generate its own 'intra-media momentum' becoming both a sign of, and contribution to, a snowball effect (Kitzinger and Reilly 1997). Editors will decide to cover an issue because 'everyone is talking about it' (Kitzinger 1998). In addition, a symbiotic relationship develops between different media outlets, whereby, for example, a documentary-maker will encourage pre-broadcast publicity through a newspaper article, and, after broadcast, the same story might be picked up by women's magazines (see, for example, the *Bella* article based on the *Homeground* documentary already mentioned).

The permeation of a story beyond straightforward news presentations can also have important implications for the *nature* and *effect* of the coverage. This is because non-news formats/outlets prioritise different production values. In addition, non-news formats are also likely to reach a different (and wider) audience and may generate a distinct type of audience engagement.

In the following section we draw on interviews with media personnel and their sources (*e.g.* press officers) in order to explore why stories about individuals from 'breast cancer families' proved so 'media-friendly'. We shall also briefly highlight the perceived advantages and disadvantages of this approach (from the perspective of journalists and of different source organisations). We then go on to examine how such media stories related to the ways in which inherited/genetic risk was discussed among ordinary women in our focus groups.

### 'Hard and soft' media values

*Views from media personnel*
To understand how the media cover genetics, it is useful to locate our findings within existing media studies theory about 'hard' and 'soft' media values. The terms 'hard' and 'soft' are commonly used by media sociologists and journalists alike to describe media output. Put simply, hard news is 'serious'; 'fact-based' coverage and soft news involves 'light' or 'human interest' stories (see Carter *et al.* 1998). Both terms relate to the subject matter, the positioning of the story, the sources used, the journalist who covers it and the implied readership.

Hard news concerns traditional front page and TV news stories which address the important issues of the day. Such reports usually rely on elite news sources (such as government departments and scientific laboratories).

They are in this sense, concerned with 'matters of State' or 'hard science', and are sometimes seen as coterminous with 'real news'. By contrast, soft news is more likely to address lower status issues (such as health or social aspects of life). It is considered more attractive to a female or youth audience and might include stories about 'abortions, lost babies, the Royal Family, fashions, the Cruft's dog show' (Schlesinger 1987: 155) or 'relationships, fashion, beauty and childcare' (Allan 1998: 132–4). In recent years however several researchers have argued that the traditional divisions between hard and soft news have become blurred. This is either seen as a process of 'dumbing down' or as a real effort to take on the public aspects of 'private domains' (*e.g.* around health and sexuality). In part such changes are certainly encouraged by media organisations' increasing attempts to pursue female readers and the youth market (see Carter *et al.* 1998, Aldridge 1994).

Several journalists interviewed for our study were quite clear that breast cancer was peculiarly 'media friendly' in part because of soft news values and the pursuit of women readers:

> [It is] a way of talking up the women's vote, if you like. Let's play the female card. Women are bound to want to read this and let's make newspaper more female friendly is the big drive. (Medical/health correspondent, broadsheet)

Breast cancer was generally identified as an easy story for any journalist, one for which he or she could be sure of editorial support. As one former medical/health correspondent explained:

> It [breast cancer] is incredibly newsworthy. It will virtually walk into a paper compared to trying to write about other forms of cancer of arguably greater social consequences. . . . You only have to go up to the news desk and say 'There is something about breast cancer' and they will say 'We will have it' and 'Go and do it'.

Although many breast cancer stories are, in media terms, newsworthy, breast cancer *genetics* has the added dimension of soft value appeal. This can be clearly seen in the nature of reporting around different elements of genetic/inherited breast cancer.

For example, the initial reporting which followed announcements of the discovery of BRCA1 and 2 was obviously informed, in part, by a hard news agenda. Coverage headlined the 'news of the day' about research 'breakthroughs' and relied on high status sources such as the Institute of Cancer Research press conference and interviews with research scientists. However, the initial TV media announcements about the genetic discoveries moved swiftly to the reactions of individuals who might benefit from these discoveries and this strategy was also adopted by the press. So, for example, a double page spread in *The Mirror* about BRCA2 juxtaposed the work of

Professor Stratton who 'beat the world to find a gene that increases women's risk of breast cancer' with the personal testimony of a young woman, Annmarie. The headline read: 'Saved by the Gene Genius: After four years of research Mike Stratton found the gene which causes breast cancer . . . two weeks later Annmarie had a blood test that changed her life' (28 July 1997). This woman tested negative for BRCA2 so decided not to proceed with a prophylactic mastectomy. The health editor responsible for this article commented that this case study was included because it allowed readers to 'understand what it meant' to have (or not have) the gene and because the story provided 'drama', prophylactic mastectomies being such a shocking operation to contemplate.

Indeed, the example of prophylactic mastectomies may even be introduced into news stories that have little to do with breast cancer per se. One broadsheet health editor we interviewed, for example, was in the process of writing a report about a new British Medical Association book on human genetics. The book, she said, 'is not at all about breast cancer', however, 'In fact I have just written a paragraph: "There are some women who face breast cancer genes and some women opt to have a mastectomy" '. She had chosen this way of introducing the issue because:

> It is quite emotive in the genetics side of it because of the prophylactic removal. It is such a dramatic thing for a woman to do but that makes it quite newsworthy. (Health Editor broadsheet)

Personal stories can put a 'human face' to the science and were seen as an accessible way of exploring social implications and personal dilemmas (a theme illustrated in most depth in *The Decision*) as well as capturing audience attention.

The attractions of breast cancer genetics as a way of making genetics 'dramatic' and 'accessible' have not gone unnoticed by those on the other side of the media presentation process: the sources. Press officers and campaigners in the field all mentioned the 'human drama' of genetics. A spokesperson for one pressure group summarised the observations of many when he commented that journalists seemed to be interested in breast cancer genetics because it allowed them to tell stories involving 'death, sex, love, motherhood and the right to choose'. We would add that inherited/genetic breast cancer can evoke powerful emotions, fear and tragedy (early death, multiple bereavement). It can disrupt or intensify relationships (sisters, mothers, daughters, lovers). It also sets the scene for secrets, discovery, and decision-making (how do you tell other members or your family? should you have prophylactic treatment?). In addition, these accounts can involve considerable narrative suspense (will she/won't she test positive?). These are all the standard characteristics of 'soft news' or even soap opera, but can be drawn upon in a wide range of media accounts (Henderson 1996a, 1996b, 1999). This is all good news for the media, but the implications may be less welcome for those seeking to promote public understanding of cancer or genetics.

*Views from source organisations and individuals*
The mobilisation of dramatic themes in 'soft' representations of inherited/genetic breast cancer provoked mixed reactions from press officers and campaigners. Responses among those we interviewed depended, in part, on their individual/organisational priorities and whether they were considering specific reports/programmes or the cumulative effects of a genre. Often the same programme would receive contradictory verdicts from different interviewees.

A common complaint against 'straight' news reporting of genetic discoveries is that science is celebrated uncritically, and social-ethical issues are ignored. By contrast some 'soft' presentations clearly allow space for exploring problematic implications and the 'messiness' of the choices to be made. This was welcomed by some of those sceptical about what they perceived to be an unrelenting discourse of progress in science reporting.

Making breast cancer genetics accessible, allowing viewers to engage in the psycho-social dynamics, and reaching a broad audience in new ways, can all also be seen as positive aspects of the human interest framing. A representative from Breast Cancer Care, for example, who collaborated with the *Peak Practice* episode discussed earlier, told us that the programme had led to a dramatic increase in calls to their telephone helpline, and commented on the number of calls from 'high risk' women who were seeking advice for the first time.

However, some of the 'soft' presentations of inherited/genetic breast cancer were criticised as distorting the 'true picture' about genetics, playing up drama over 'fact' and focusing on tragedy and pathos. Wendy Watson has extensive experience as a media source. She has frequently presented her own personal experience and is now an activist in the field (*e.g.* promoting information to women with a family history of the disease). She expressed mixed feelings about the media. Although praising *The Decision* and many newspaper reporters, she complains that some journalists tried to play up the terror of her experience. 'One magazine wrote this absolutely vile article . . . They managed to find this glum picture, you know, this stony face, and then: "So scared of breast cancer I had my breasts removed" '. She told us how another women's magazine published a letter purporting to be from her which totally misrepresented her experience and described how some journalists tried to manipulate her story while they were interviewing her. One women's magazine journalist, for example, was clearly influenced by previous media representations of Breast Cancer Family Trees (showing those with cancer genes as black circles and squares). This journalist tried to persuade Wendy Watson to represent her own story in these terms:[3]

> [One] writer wanted me to say 'I looked at the paper and I saw all these black circles and then I decided that [prophylactic mastectomy] was what

I must do'. But it wasn't like that. [The journalist] said: 'I really like this black circle business'. I said: 'well, I never saw any black circles, you know, you can't quote me on black circles'.

Even without such obvious manipulation of 'first person' accounts, the coverage of inherited/genetic risk was viewed with concern by some cancer organisations. Charities sometimes criticised representations for being unclear about the nature of inherited risk, and the sheer extent of attention to genetic causes was also problematised by some:

> A lot of people think if they've got some dim and distant relative who has had breast cancer then it's a sure fire thing that they're also going to get breast cancer . . . Breast cancers at the moment have got to be genetic breast cancers. I think largely the media are responsible for that. (Breast cancer charity representative)

Clearly, judgements about the impact of different representations are not straightforward. Each of the speakers we have quoted draws on different types of experience and feedback from women. In the final section of this chapter we shall add our own reflections to this debate by drawing on our focus group data to explore how women talked about inherited/genetic risk and how they related to the media.

## A brief look at women's understandings of genetic/inherited risk

Our 25 focus group discussions with 143 ordinary women confirmed observations made by those working with members of the public on a day-to-day basis. Research participants tended to over-estimate the role of genetics in the aetiology of breast cancer and were often unclear about the nature of genetic risk.

During the course of the research sessions, participants were asked to estimate the proportion of women with breast cancer who had developed it because of a family history of the disease. Most women opted for a figure over 50 per cent. In only five groups did anyone offer estimates lower than 20 per cent.

The importance attributed to family history was also evident in the way that women discussed their own risk. Women with just one relative, or a couple of elderly relatives, who had breast cancer, sometimes gave this as a reason for feeling at risk. Others, with no known family history, interpreted this to mean that there was very little risk of them contracting the disease: 'I don't think there's a risk of it because it's not in my family' (Group 9); 'I associate it mostly with hereditary type things and I know I haven't got a family history at all, so I'm sort of quite complacent that way' (Group 13); 'My awareness of it [breast cancer] is purely a genetic thing' (Group 18).

The emphasis placed on inherited risk cannot, of course, be entirely attributed to specific media coverage. Other factors come into play including personal experience and questioning about family history by doctors as well as pre-existing cultural ideas about the importance of inheritance (Davison *et al.* 1992) and the increasing overall cultural 'geneticisation' of illness (Nelkin and Lindee 1995). However, the key role of the media in informing women's assessments was clearly evident in the way in which women referred to the media to explain and justify their emphasis on family history. The sheer quantity of reporting about inherited/genetic risk was one factor. 'It must be high', declared one woman 'because such a big deal is made of it' (Group 7). 'I would have said more than 60 per cent of breast cancers were due to inherited risk', commented another, 'It's certainly the one that's pushed the most' (Group 1). 'I think whenever I've heard of people having it' observed a third research participant, 'it seems to run in the family' (Group 12).

The nature of the coverage, particularly the human interest coverage, was also key. Women spoke at length about magazine articles, documentaries, fictional representations and chat shows. The focus was on the dramatised personal accounts of 'breast cancer families'. It was these, rather than routine news reports about genetic discoveries (or patenting or testing debates), which had made most impression. Indeed, in several groups it became clear that people were unaware that any 'breast cancer genes' had been discovered and only three women mentioned a news report (press or TV) as informing their sense of inherited risk, and one of these women explicitly stated that it was: 'one of those sorts of human interest stories at the end' (Group 18).

Not only were such human interest stories raised spontaneously in most of the group discussions but it was also clear that they had often generated conversation between people *prior* to the research session. In addition, even if the women could not specify where they had seen the story (and people do not necessarily correctly attribute their source) they often had quite vivid memories which allowed us to identify the type (if not the precise source) of account to which they were referring. Research participants often, for example, recalled visual images such as family photographs or diagrams of the family tree. They also could often described the narrative structure of the accounts. The following quote is typical of the way research participants recalled media stories about inherited/genetic risk:

> They took their family tree all the way back and right through their families. The amount of women that had died early from [breast cancer] was heartbreaking. [. . .] [One woman] was in her 20s, they both had wee kiddies, and they were both going to have to do that [have prophylactic mastectomies]. They were heartbroken but they had made the decision (Group 5).

Stories about women from 'high risk families' had made a profound impression on them, women said, because of the youth of those affected: 'they were quite young, so, that's the one that sticks out' (Group 6). Such stories were also memorable because: 'the fear just came across so much' (Group 25); 'It can blight a family' (Group 13); 'It seems such a drastic thing for any woman to do' (Group 24). Some research participants recalled the stories because they were 'so weird' ('I thought how could they do that to themselves, just in case. That seemed horrific, like self-mutilation' Group 11). Often it was also clear that research participants had empathised with women's dilemmas: 'That must be a terrible thing, if you know there's nothing wrong with you, to go in and be operated on, you know, healthy breasts' (Group 3); 'They chose mastectomies . . . Imagine having to make that choice' (Group 18).

We shall be doing further analysis to explore women's understandings of inherited/genetic risk. Here, we simply wish to highlight the fact that human interest stories were the types of media coverage which generated conversation, thought and reflection and were most vividly recalled. Some of the women who could reconstruct the images and narrative structures of such coverage in great depth knew very little about genetics (*e.g.* being unaware of how risks were calculated, and even, in some cases, being unaware that any 'gene' had been identified at all). It seems that human interest stories or personalised accounts may convey ideas about inherited risk independently from knowledge about research discoveries and genetic 'facts'.

**Conclusion**

This chapter points to the ways in which genetic 'discoveries' have been explored through diverse media coverage. We have highlighted the media values which may promote certain types of stories and presentational styles over others. We have also suggested ways in which this influences public understandings. These preliminary findings have implications both for predicting how coverage of genetics might evolve and for developing future media research and intervention strategies.

*Implications for predicting media coverage of genetics*
We have focused on coverage of breast cancer; the chapter suggests, however, patterns in how *other* inherited/genetic risks might be represented. Clearly, genetic risk appeals to a broad range of media because it is about inheritance and family relationships (as well as uncertainty, tragedy, and decisions). It offers the potential to explore the dilemmas of *The Decision* when *Living in the Shadow* or exploit the drama of 'a family curse'. Such stories can contain elements of the most popular hospital drama and family complications of *Dynasty* proportions. Genetics per se will thus be of interest to a broad range of media personnel working in diverse formats and outlets, particularly for those working with a 'soft' agenda.

At the same time it is important to acknowledge that coverage of any particular genetic risk will vary depending, for a start on the scientific/policy context for that particular gene. For example, coverage will be influenced by progress not only in identifying a gene, but also in developing a test for it, and, perhaps, intervention procedures. Such developments will shift media attention onto the dilemmas raised for individuals. Our earlier research suggested that the traditional news media are not well adapted for considering the potential social implications of on-going scientific research in any consistent and sustained way (see Kitzinger and Reilly 1997). Such considerations have traditionally been addressed within futuristic, science fiction type genres. However, once the media can access 'real people' actually facing choices around testing and treatment then attention will increase and diffuse into a wider range of media outlets.

Coverage of any particular genetic risk will also vary depending on the social context and characteristics with which that gene is associated. Media attention will be influenced by questions such as: who is this gene supposed to affect; how, when, with what consequences? In the case study presented here we have shown how coverage of breast cancer genetics was influenced by the widespread nature of breast cancer and its impact on young women, combined with media efforts to target female audiences. Elsewhere, we have also argued that coverage was influenced by the social acceptability of breast cancer and celebrity alignment with the disease, as well as the particular cultural fascination and horror associated with mastectomy (see Saywell *et al.* 1999). Such specifics need to be taken into account when considering the media profile of any particular gene. Not all genes will have the same media appeal. For example, genes concerned with behaviour, such as the so-called 'crime gene', may be more controversial than genes associated with ill health, and different types of coverage will be generated in relation to the 'gay gene' or the gene for Alzheimer's (Kitzinger and Reilly 1997, Conrad 1998, Cunningham-Burley *et al.* 1998).

*Implications for research strategies*
The data reported here demonstrate that it is insufficient only to examine straightforward health/science reporting. It is crucial to include human interest representations and 'soft' outlets such as women's weekly magazines. This is vital if we are to establish a full picture of the representations actually reaching and influencing the public.

Our study shows that different formats and outlets may prioritise different themes and that some issues (such as prophylactic mastectomies) translate across different formats/outlets, while others (such as the patenting debate) may not. This has implications for the quantity, but also for the nature, of representation. The process of translation between different formats and outlets may reiterate particular representations, but may also shift them. On the one hand there is considerable overlap between 'soft' and 'hard' media agendas. On the other hand 'soft' reporting may introduce new problems and new potential. Soft reporting might be more accessible than hard reporting but it might mask scientific information behind emotive stories. It might be better at addressing the psycho-social aspects of an issue, but may also distort these into a series of clichés. A soap opera story-line can reach out to a new constituency, encouraging people to seek further information, but it can also heighten fear or complacency. Detailed attention to specific representations, as well as examination of cumulative influence, would therefore be needed to explore which programmes and stories have which effects under what circumstances.

What our research does suggest, however, is that soft values may actually invert many of the values of 'hard news' (as traditionally defined). Where hard values privilege high status official sources, soft values prioritise 'ordinary' women's accounts (however these might be twisted in the process). Where hard values lead reporters to abhor uncertainty (preferring clear-cut 'breakthroughs' or controversy around sharply opposing positions), it is precisely uncertainty which may provide the drama in a personal account or fictional presentation. Where hard news about scientific discoveries often relies heavily on scientific press releases and may ignore potential problems, soft presentations and fictional accounts may explore the shades of grey. As news reporting is increasingly seen to adopt 'soft values' it is vital to understand the implications of this shift. It is important to engage with diverse formats and outlets (as researchers and campaigners) in ways which do not dismiss 'soft' reporting as inherently weaker, without due consideration of its potential as well as its limitations.

In conclusion, as the science develops and as social researchers, practitioners, the media and the public become increasingly interested in the social and psychological aspects of genetics, attention to a diversity of cultural representation and 'soft' forms is particularly important. It may be here that new problems with representation might be identified. However, it may also be here that opportunities for debate and communication might be found.

## Acknowledgements

This project is funded by the NHS executive R & D initiative. We also wish to thank colleagues at the Glasgow University Media Research Unit: Cherise Saywell, Liz Beattie and Greg Philo, as well as the interviewees and focus group participants who have contributed to this research.

## Notes

1   British newspapers are traditionally refereed to as 'tabloid' or 'broadsheet', which technically relates to the paper size. However, these terms also relate to readership, influence and news values. Thus broadsheet signifies 'serious, high

income readership, lower sales but more influence' (papers such as *The Times*). Tabloid papers divide into two groups: the 'mid-market' *Daily Mail* and *Daily Express* which cater to those with a middle-income and *The Sun* and *The Daily Mirror* aimed primarily at low-income readership. These last two are the top selling newspapers in Britain (see Aldridge 1994 for more detail).

2   The age of a woman was usually only mentioned as a risk factor in an implicit way. Press articles which contained statements such as 'she was only 33 so it was a shock to have cancer' were coded as referencing age as a risk factor.

3   Not all women's magazines adopt the same approach. *Good Housekeeping*, for example was frequently referred to by cancer charity press officers and focus group participants as an important conduit for high quality, factual health information. The Health Editor of *Good Housekeeping*, explained that her position as 'health editor', combined with the production team's perceptions of the magazines' readership, influenced how genetics was covered: 'We're quite unusual amongst women's magazines in that [. . .] we actually have a specialised health editor whereas women's magazines have health-and-beauty editors so they tend to do less research. But *Good Housekeeping* does normally cover the research side of health. we're very conscious that our readers are at the age where they need health coverage that enables them to make decisions, to make choices. [. . .] They want information that they can take down to the doctor's surgery and they're not just interested in fluff or psychological side so we do try and give them quite strong medical information, stuff they can use'.

# References

Aldridge, M. (1994) *Making Social Work News*. London: Routledge.

Allan, S. (1998) (En)gendering the truth politics of news discourse. In Carter, C., Branston, G. and Allan, S. (eds) *News, Gender and Power*. London: Routledge.

Carter, C., Branston, G. and Allan, S. (eds) (1998) *News, Gender and Power*. London: Routledge.

Chapman, S. and Lupton, D. (1994) *The Fight for Public Health*. London: British Medical Journal Publishing.

Conrad, P. (1998) Public eyes and private genes, *Social Problems*, 44, 2, 139–54.

Cunningham-Burley, S., Kerr, A. and Amos, A. (1998) *The Social and Cultural Impact on the New Genetics*, final reports to the ESRC.

Davison, C., Frankel, S. and Davey-Smith, G. (1992) The limits of lifestyle: re-assessing fatalism in popular culture of illness prevention, *Social Science and Medicine*, 34, 675–85.

Easton, D.F., Narod, S.A., Ford, D. and Steel, M. (1994) The genetic epidemiology of BRCA1, *Lancet*, 344, 761.

Entwhistle, V. (1995) Reporting research in medical journals and newspapers, *British Medical Journal*, 310: 920–3.

Friedman, M., Dunwoody, S. and Rogers, C. (eds) (1986) *Scientists and Journalists: Reporting Science as News*. New York: Free Press.

Henderson, L. (1996a) *Incest in Brookside: Audience Responses to the Jordache Story*. London: Channel 4 Television.

Henderson, L. (1996b) Selling suffering: mental illness and media values. In Philo, G. (ed) *The Media and Mental Distress*. Harlow: Addison Wesley and Longman.

Henderson, L. (1999) Making serious soaps: sensitive issues in TV drama. In Philo, G. (ed) *The Media and Mental Distress*. Harlow: Addison Wesley and Longman.

Hilgartner, S. and Bosk, C. (1988) The rise and fall of social problems, *American Journal of Sociology*, 94, 1, 53–78.

Karpf, A. (1988) *Doctoring the Media*. London: Routledge.

Kerr, A., Cunningham Burley, S. and Amos, A. (1998) Drawing the line: an analysis of people's discussion about the new genetics, *Public Understanding of Science*, 7, 13–33.

Kitzinger, J. (1999) Researching risk and the media, *Health, Risk and Society*, 1, 1, 55–69.

Kitzinger, J. (1998) The gender politics of news production. In Carter, C., Branston, G. and Allan, S. (eds) *News, Gender and Power*. London: Routledge.

Kitzinger, J. and Reilly, J. (1997) The rise and fall of risk reporting, *European Journal of Communication* 12, 3, 319–50.

Miller, D. (1995) Introducing the 'gay gene', *Public Understanding of Science*, 4, 269–84.

Miller, D., Kitzinger, J., Williams, K. and Beharrell, P. (1998) *The Circuit of Mass Communication: Media Strategies, Representation and Audience Reception in the AIDS Crisis*. London: Sage.

Moyer, A., Greener, S., Beauvais, J. and Salovey, P., (1995) Accuracy of health research reported in the popular press, *Health Communication*, 7, 2, 147–61.

Nelkin, D. (1996) An uneasy relationship: the tensions between medicine and the media, *Lancet*, 347, 1600–3.

Nelkin, D. and Lindee, S. (1995) *The DNA Mystique*. New York: Freeman.

Peters, H., P. (1995) The interaction of journalists and scientific experts, *Media, Culture and Society*, 17, 31–48.

Philo, G. (ed) (1999) *Message Received*. Harlow: Addison, Wesley and Longman.

Richards, M., Hallowell, N., Green, J., Murton, F. and Statham, H. (1995) Counselling families with hereditary breast and ovarian cancer, *Journal of Genetic Counselling*, 4, 3, 219–31.

Saywell, C., Henderson, L. and Beattie, L. (1999) Sexualised illness: the newsworthy body in media representations of breast cancer. In Potts, L. (ed) *Ideologies of Breast Cancer*. London: Macmillan.

Schlesinger, P. (1987) *Putting Reality Together: BBC News*. London: Routledge.

Turney, J. (1998) *Frankenstein's Footsteps: Science, Genetics and Popular Culture*. Yale: Yale University Press.

Wellcome Trust (1998) *Public Perspectives on Human Cloning*. London: The Wellcome Trust.

Wilkie, T. (1991) Does science get the press it deserves? *International Journal of Science Education*, 13, 5, 575–81.

Wooster, R., Neuhausen, S.L., Mangion, J., Quirk, Y., Ford, D. and Collins, N. (1994) Localisation of a breast cancer susceptibility gene BRCA2 to chromosome 13q 12–13, *Science*, 265, 2088–90.

# II: The Social Meanings of Genetics

# Waiting for the cure: mapping the social relations of human gene therapy research

*Alan Stockdale*

## Introduction

Public participation is often proclaimed to be an important component in a wise process of biomedical technology development. The policy discussions surrounding somatic cell gene therapy, a set of therapeutic strategies based on the transfer of genetic material into the non-reproductive cells of patients, are claimed to be a shining example. Bayertz *et al.*, for example, state that:

> no other form of therapy in the history of medicine has undergone such an intensive process of public debate, examination and appraisal before its application as somatic cell gene therapy. . . . The introduction of somatic cell gene therapy may be regarded as a model example of a new relationship between biomedical innovation and the public: as a model example of regulated scientific and technical progress (1994: 466).

It is true that during the 1980s there was extensive debate by government appointed groups and groups within key government agencies that resulted in a series of reports and guidelines that legitimated the start of clinical gene therapy trials in 1990 (see Fletcher 1990, Murray 1990, Walters 1991). However, there is little evidence to suggest that patients with diseases targeted by gene therapy research, much less the public, have participated in 'public debate', or that they are well informed about gene therapy. This chapter, based on a study of the development of genetic therapies for cystic fibrosis (CF) in the United States, will identify aspects of the research process that are problematic for some patients and their families, and factors that have limited their active participation in the research process. These factors have resulted in the pursuit of a research agenda with little consideration or understanding of its consequences for people living with CF.

## Study approach

Sociological work on the public understanding of genetics has largely focused, quite appropriately, on the contexts in which consumers appropriate genetic knowledge. This approach has been formulated in response to professional groups' framing of the public as undifferentiated, ignorant of genetics, and in need of education (Durant *et al.* 1996, Kerr *et al.* 1997, 1998, Turney 1995). While professional ignorance of 'the public' has also been an interesting aspect of this type of analysis, this approach is in danger of remaining trapped in the original binary framing. This framing might usefully be exploded into a more complex mapping of the cultural constructions and social relationships that span the numerous intersecting contexts in which genetics is an important feature. The complexities and tensions inherent in the relationships within and between professional groups— physicians, researchers, journalists, professional fundraisers—have an important bearing on the public presentation of genetic technologies.

Critical to understanding the conflicts and discontinuities inherent in the cultures surrounding genetic research, is a sociology of cultural worlds (Young 1982). Particularly important in this respect are the ongoing struggles of speciality groups, institutions, and consumer groups for legitimacy and the power to exert control over medical practice and scientific research (Hahn and Kleinman 1983). A key element by which power is extended is through control over the legitimisation and circulation of knowledge. Asymmetries in access to media and various other public and private forums are therefore an important element that underlies and sustains differentials in power between groups and discontinuities in their social worlds (Hannerz 1992). Consumers are often in a weak position, not necessarily having the means to necessitate their active participation in the work of other key groups (but see Epstein 1995).

The work presented here is based on an approach that was developed to map an extended network of beliefs and relationships (see Marcus 1995). This involved a trade-off in depth for breadth; however, the aim of the research was to identify tensions and contradictions that will be explored by more systematic and focused research in the future. The more specific goal of my research was to map roughly the activities and perspectives of an extended network of groups spread across medical, research, and other institutional settings, and lay out a range of issues of concern to people with CF in the context of gene therapy research.

To accomplish this mapping, data were drawn from a wide range of sources between 1994 and 1998 to gain a broad sense of the relationships between key groups. Forty interviews were conducted with physicians, researchers, parents of children with CF, adults with CF, representatives of charities and consumer organisations, employees and representatives of the biotechnology industry, and others. Interviewees were selected on the basis of convenience, often through snowball sampling. A substantial source of data was Cystic-L, an e-mail discussion list on the Internet devoted to the discussion of topics related to CF. This list was founded in early 1994 and by 1996 had approximately 600 subscribers, mostly American adults with CF and parents of children with CF. More than 15,000 e-mail messages, most of which were sent before 1997, were analysed. (Note that in the following text participants in Cystic-L and interviewees are identified by a common numbering scheme as the two groups overlap.) Data were also taken from scientific and medical journals, biotechnology trade publications, government publications and reports, consumer newsletters, and a wide range of popular news magazines and daily newspapers. Conferences and other meetings were another important source of data, including CF gene therapy conferences, national and international CF conferences, CF conferences organised by consumer groups, and hospital events for CF patients and their parents.

**Marketing and misunderstanding**

The development and deployment of somatic cell gene therapy for serious diseases has been assumed to be relatively unproblematic. Yet, possible benefits, whether measured in hope or improved control over disease, should not obscure the difficulties gene therapy research poses for populations with diseases targeted for gene therapy. Gene therapy is not readily assimilated to any easily understood model of therapeutic action and poses considerable problems for understanding. It should be borne in mind that many physicians and a large section of the public have difficulty understanding even basic genetic concepts (Durant *et al.* 1996, Hofman *et al.* 1993, Richards 1996, Turney 1995).

Gene therapy has the aura of a miracle technology whereas the reality is more ordinary. The first decade of human gene therapy research has so far demonstrated that there are no quick solutions to developing systems that are capable of delivering genetic material to the correct cells, in sufficient quantity to have a lasting therapeutic effect, without toxic side-effects resulting from either the vector used to carry the genetic material or over-expression of the gene product. In fact, the term gene therapy is a misnomer at the present time given the lack of demonstrated therapies. The large number of clinical trials in recent years is also somewhat misleading. Unlike more traditional pharmaceuticals, which succeed or fail in clinical tests, 'failed' gene therapy trials merely feed a cycle of tinkering and further clinical trials to produce a delivery method that may eventually work safely and effectively. As Orkin and Motulsky (1995) note, 'although widely referred to as "clinical trials", gene transfer protocols to date are in truth smallscale clinical experiments'. Even if successful, many of the therapies under development would not be cures in the strict sense of the term. They are likely to have limited and variable effects, might have to be readministered at regular intervals and used in combination with other therapies. This, at least, is the likely scenario for a disease such as CF. The illusion that the effects of gene therapy will be more fundamental is sustained by the mistaken belief that current strategies 'correct' the underlying genetic error. Although rarely discussed, gene therapy is also likely to be expensive, particularly for diseases like CF that have relatively small populations, a not insignificant issue given the ongoing crisis in access to affordable healthcare.

The miracle technology aura of gene therapy was initially fed by research hype and extensive, but uncritical, media coverage. After the first clinical gene therapy experiment in 1990 and accompanying the rapid expansion of clinical experimentation, the media were awash with hype, pronouncements of a medical revolution brought about by molecular research, and predictions that cures for previously incurable genetic diseases would be available in a few years (*e.g.* Maugh 1990, 1992, Purvis 1992, Rensberger 1992). This enthusiasm for gene therapy was fed by researchers and their supporters. At the time there were many new gene therapy companies looking for financial backing when venture capital funding for biotechnology was relatively scarce as a result of a slow economy and the threat of major health care reform. By 1995, as research failed to sustain the predictions of medical breakthroughs, the media, in many cases the same media outlets that had previously proclaimed the coming of a medical revolution, now declared gene therapy a failure (*e.g.* Gorman 1995, Palca 1995, Southwick 1995).

In late 1995 the National Institutes of Health (NIH) released a report on gene therapy that was critical of the rush to clinical trials, poor experimental design, the lack of basic research, and redundant research efforts (Orkin and Motulsky 1995). In their report Orkin and Motulsky argued that the hype surrounding gene therapy research was damaging the credibility of the field:

> Overselling of the results of laboratory and clinical studies by investigators and their sponsors—be they academic, federal, or industrial—has led to the mistaken and widespread perception that gene therapy is further developed and more successful than it actually is. Such inaccurate portrayals threaten confidence in the integrity of the field and may ultimately hinder progress toward successful application of gene therapy to human disease (1995)

They argued that none of the gene therapy experiments had as yet clearly demonstrated efficacy. Considerable effort would need to be devoted to understanding the underlying pathology of target diseases and to the development of improved delivery methods for gene therapy to become successful in treating disease. Gene therapy, they argued, was a technology in its infancy and required time to fulfill its potential.

Orkin and Motulsky's analysis of the media publicity surrounding gene therapy was echoed by some other researchers (*e.g.* Friedmann 1996); however, gene therapy researchers are divided on this issue: some have embraced the media and others have shunned it. A couple of years earlier, Richard Mulligan (1993: 931), a gene therapy researcher at Harvard University, had warned about the 'fervor to introduce gene therapy into the clinic' and the assessment of research in the media. But the industry has often found it difficult to forgo clinical trials and shun publicity, as hinted by a researcher at a biotechnology company:

... I think what has, what we missed perhaps at the beginning is that we should really concentrate on the basic principles and try to, try to see what the basic mechanisms of all this are. And what we did and what we always do when a new field emerges of whatever kind is that we rush to the clinic . . . and just to make it to the front page of the *Science* or into *The Wall Street Journal* now, and that has consistently turned out to be disastrous. It is actually really sad because we should know better (interviewee 30, 1995).

Whatever their other intentions, commercial pressures on the biotechnology industry often drive clinical research and relationships with the media.

Since there is not unlimited public funding for research, gene therapy research has initially often been done by researchers at medical schools in partnerships with biotechnology companies. Many of these companies are small and lack an income stream from existing products, and therefore need to generate financial support through venture capital or partnerships with pharmaceuticals (Hillman *et al.* 1996). Publicity plays an important role in this process, a point put bluntly by Alan Smith, head of gene therapy research at the biotechnology company Genzyme, who stated in reaction to the Orkin and Motulsky Report:

... there is a lot of basic research to be done, and it doesn't help to be hyping the field. On the other hand, part of running a business is getting funded, and hype wouldn't be unheard of. The biotech industry was accused of that from the beginning (quoted in Brown 1996:1)

In practice, therefore, the economics of research makes it unlikely that biotechnology will be conducted outside the glare of the media, although a moderating factor now may be the rapid acquisition of many American biotechnology companies with gene therapy programmes by European pharmaceuticals (Martin and Thomas 1996).

Another concern expressed by some researchers is the impact of hype on patients and families. Orkin and Motulsky (1995) state that 'patients, their families, and health providers may make unwise decisions regarding treatment alternatives, holding out for cures that they mistakenly believe are "just round the corner" '. Others point to the emotional impact of raised and dashed hopes on families struggling with life-threatening diseases. Theodore Friedmann, a pioneer of gene therapy research, writes:

Some gene therapy papers, manuscripts and funding applications have in the past sent, and at times still send, overstated messages of successful *therapy*, even in the obvious absence of convincing evidence of clinical benefit. No matter how well-intentioned, such hyperbole and exaggerated expectations can be a cruel disservice to patients and their families (Friedmann 1996: 145, emphasis in the original).

As little research has been done on these issues, it is difficult to evaluate the broad impact of gene therapy publicity in this regard.

Better education of patients and physicians is sometimes cited as a solution. Kenneth Culver, another pioneer of gene therapy research, points out that physicians need to be in a position where they can discuss gene therapy experiments with their patients:

> I think that one of the fundamental efforts should be a broad-based education campaign that explains the possibilities and limitations of gene therapy. After reading that the gene for their disease has been cloned, most patients are shocked when we tell them that there is a lot more involved than cloning the gene. There is a tremendous level of ignorance in the general population. . . . I think it has been beneficial to report on new genetic discoveries in a prominent way. The biggest deficiency is that, in general, the medical community is not prepared to discuss the information with patients (Hillman *et al.* 1996: 1142).

While some of this anxiety concerning the lack of education is undoubtedly occasioned by genuine concern for patients and their families, it is also related to the potential long-term impact of hype on research programmes (Orkin and Motulsky 1995).

There is reason to treat pronouncements by researchers on the need for public education with some scepticism (Kerr *et al.* 1997). Assertions that the solution lies in more lay or physician education makes the lack of knowledge possessed by others the problem. Implicit in this is the conceptualisation of education as a top-down process from researchers to others, a course of action that conveniently recreates the authoritative position of the researcher, who now becomes part of the solution to the problem instead of part of the cause. As we shall see, it seems equally reasonable to argue that researchers are as much in need of education about patient concerns as patients are in need of being provided with a realistic understanding of gene therapy research and what it might accomplish.

Finally, it is worth noting some deficiencies in the two groups that have a role in ensuring human subjects in gene therapy trials are informed and protected: NIH's Recombinant DNA Advisory Committee (RAC) and Institutional Review Boards (IRBs). The RAC has been the most visible forum for consumer participation, although this has been quite limited and there have been ongoing struggles to limit its role. As for IRBs, it has been widely argued that most are not up to the task of protecting human subjects in this context as they lack access to the expertise, both professional and lay, necessary to perform the task adequately (Office of Inspector General 1998). Neither the RAC (Zallen 1996: 795) nor IRBs (Office of Inspector General 1998: 8–9) have adequate mechanisms for evaluating performance because little or no feedback is solicited from human subjects and their families. Tellingly, what little is known about the experience of gene therapy research subjects comes from critical accounts published in the newsletters of consumer groups (Claassen 1998, Gustavson 1997, *cf.* Claassen with Recombinant DNA Advisory Committee 1994).

## The cystic fibrosis experience

The experience and relationships in the CF case are a striking example of the lack of consumer involvement in the research process. CF is a recessive genetic disease that affects the lungs, digestive system, and other organs. Accumulated damage to the lungs resulting from opportunistic bacterial infection usually causes death in early to mid-adulthood. The gene that causes CF, the cystic fibrosis transmembrane conductance regulator (CFTR) gene, was discovered in 1989. The discovery was a major break-through; however, the pathogenesis of CF has proved to be complex and is still incompletely understood.

The CFTR gene was discovered just as clinical gene therapy research was becoming a reality and CF rapidly became a major focus of gene therapy research. A number of laboratory experiments quickly demonstrated that it was possible to express the gene in cell lines and in animal models. The first CF gene therapy clinical trials were approved in late 1992 and the first trials conducted early in 1993. In the United States, at least eight biotechnology companies, many formed in the 1990s, have been actively engaged in CF gene therapy research, usually with academic partners.

The Cystic Fibrosis Foundation (CFF), an organisation founded in the late 1950s by parents and physicians to promote research, awareness and better care for people with CF, has played an important role in the promotion of gene therapy research. In the 1980s the CFF actively sought to attract the best researchers by concentrating funds in a few key research centres and extending the period of grant support. It also transformed itself at this time into an efficient fundraiser. By 1995 the CFF was generating $100 million a year, about a quarter of this going to research, or about half as much as NIH devotes to CF research. The CFF jointly funds projects in conjunction with NIH, including the NIH's designated gene therapy research centres. The CFF also functions as an important mediator, linking researchers at medical schools and biotechnology companies, and facilitating relationships between these groups and the NIH, the Food and Drug Administration (FDA), and legislators. It runs two important annual conferences: the North American Cystic Fibrosis Conference (NACF), attended by thousands of medical professionals and researchers from all over the world, and the Williamsburg Conference, a small meeting of invited researchers from academia and industry, and key officers at the FDA and the NIH. The CFF also plays an important lobbying role, promoting and protecting NIH funding, as well as protection of financial incentives for development of drugs to treat rare diseases, patenting, control over pharmaceutical pricing, and other matters of importance to researchers and the biotechnology industry that might be impacted by legislation. In addition to all the above, the CFF sets standards and provides accreditation for nearly all the CF Clinical Centers in the United States.

The discovery of the CFTR gene and the initial CF gene therapy experiments were accompanied by extensive and positive publicity. For example, in 1990 the *Los Angeles Times* published the following on the successful laboratory expression of CFTR:

> The new findings announced Thursday in articles in the journals *Cell* and *Nature* suggest it may be possible within a few years to cure the disease either by replacing the defective gene with a healthy one through gene therapy, by delivering an intact protein to the diseased cells or by the development of new drugs. 'We're not talking decades, we're talking years, a few years', said Robert J. Beall, medical director of the Cystic Fibrosis Foundation. 'We're very excited' (Maugh 1990: 1).

Note the use of the words 'replacement' and 'cure' and the short predicted time frame. These were recurrent features of media reporting on CF gene therapy research in the early 1990s. In 1992 *Time Magazine* proclaimed: 'thanks to a series of breakthroughs, doctors are closing in on a cure for cystic fibrosis' (Purvis 1992: 60) and the *Los Angeles Times* quoted a prominent CF gene therapy researcher as saying: 'I have no doubt that if we were to [use the altered virus] now in a person with cystic fibrosis that we could . . . reverse the abnormalities in the lung' (Maugh 1992: 1). These are typical examples of the media coverage at that time. The CFF was also mass mailing charity solicitations—which often go to families living with CF—that made pitches like the following one from 1994:

> Scientists now have the key to unlock the final secrets of cystic fibrosis. We need to keep the momentum going until we can take this discovery to the next step—the cure itself. It will take a few more years and millions of dollars. But, like polio in the 1950s, someday CF will no longer threaten children's lives.

The reference to threatened children is a standard, if problematic, feature of charity solicitations and media stories (Anonymous 1993, Friedmann 1996). The slogan on the letterhead of this solicitation read: 'We are fighting a child-killer and winning'.

None of the statements made about cures is remotely close to an accurate portrayal of CF gene therapy research in the 1990s. The word cure is used frequently by researchers, journalists, and others, although the applicability of the word in this context is questionable. As one CF physician commented:

Look at what it means to a patient. If I talk about a cure what do you think I'm talking about? And people say, 'Like an injection. You give me a shot of something and I'm rid of my CF. I don't have to come to the doctor, I don't have to take medications, and I don't have to see you guys again—it goes away'. . . . When people talk about a cure for CF they are talking about fixing the cellular mechanism . . . which will require refixing and it's not going to affect the gastrointestinal side, or infertility. By definition talking about a cure is really inappropriate (interviewee 29, 1995).

None of the CF gene therapy research protocols developed so far involve gene replacement or repair. None of them, if they worked, would be a cure in the sense that a patient would be free of CF. Nor will CF gene therapy research in any form repair lung and other tissues that have been damaged as a result of the disease, although this is rarely mentioned. The physician just quoted also made the following observation:

Biotech has to create hype for investment. The problem is that the hype they generate is in the public domain. It is in the *New York Times*, *The Economist*. . . . It is very public information and there is a lack of interpretation as that message is communicated from one group to another so that it is meaningful to the group who need to be addressed. The trouble is that medical and patient communities are reading that information and often for the patients there is no interpretation (interviewee 29, 1995).

The difference between the physicians and patients is of course that the physicians attend conferences, have easy access to the medical literature, and may in some cases even be working with researchers conducting clinical trials. They have some context in which to make sense of the hype.

The CFF, like many medical charities, is also caught in a publicity dilemma. It depends on volunteers to help raise money, often family members of those living with the disease, and the generosity of corporations and the general public. Improbable predictions of imminent breakthroughs coupled with the exaggerated statements of the consequences of the disease for innocent children makes for an effective pitch. However, time has run out on most of the predictions of a cure made in the early 1990s and the representation of CF as a child-killer plays loosely with the truth. Eighty per cent of people with CF survive into adulthood and there are increasing numbers of people living into their 30s and beyond (Cystic Fibrosis Foundation 1997). These representations have consequences for people living with CF. They can give a false sense of hope, distress parents, and alienate adults with the disease.

The frustrations experienced by some patients and their families do not have a public outlet as it has been difficult for them to organise independently. All they have in common is CF, they are a small and dispersed group, and one of the only venues in which they regularly meet is one they do their best to avoid, the clinical setting. And within the CFF, consumers' roles have been largely limited to those of fundraisers and cheerleaders in support of the CFF's research agenda. In recent years the Internet has changed this situation somewhat as an e-mail list devoted to CF, Cystic-L, has become an important forum for sharing knowledge, experiences, and opinions, although limited largely to people living with CF.

Research publicity, gene therapy research, and the role of the CFF have been regular and controversial topics on Cystic-L. On the representation of people with CF in publicity materials, a mother of a newly diagnosed child commented:

> I went to [my local CFF] chapter annual meeting about 10 days ago because it was held so close to where I live. They played this tear-jerking video of babies with CF and as a newcomer, frankly, it really wrenched me. I spent most of the morning wiping my eyes, feeling sorry for myself and wondering if it gets any better. . . . We are still reeling from the diagnosis (participant 11, 1995).

Some adults feel their medical and personal needs have been further marginalised—most adults with CF are treated by paediatricians—by the promotion of gene therapy. Some adults are divided in their opinions, wanting to support gene therapy research, but unhappy about the way research has been promoted to the exclusion of other needs. As one woman commented:

> I have to say that I agree that the purpose of the CFF is a noble and important one. But I have to add that their search for a cure will not help me or many of my friends with CF. My only hope is a transplant. . . . I don't mean to be gloom and doom, but I do think the CFF has [been and] is guilty of playing up research advances for the sake of raking in more dough (participant 50, 1995).

Others, like the next man, are less charitable:

> At times I get the feeling from the Foundation that they want us AWCF [Adults with CF] to just 'fade' away so as not to harm their pathetic fund raising campaigns. Yes, pathetic. We are not all little cute children, sure to die if you (the public) don't send in donations. The Foundation's almost total neglect in aiding PWCF [People with CF] in our day-to-day lives is criminal (participant 51, 1995).

Although the people who participate on this list have frequently been critical of the lack of support for those living with CF, there are people, like this adult woman with CF, who support the CFF's focus on gene therapy research:

I support CFF's rationale for directing all funds to research because this is where we all need the most help and where we can benefit the most . . . there are many children and adults older than me who are living with CF and will benefit from gene therapy one day. The logic behind this research is so good, it is bound to work. It will just take more time and good science and money. . . . I believe in the mission of the CFF and believe that, to be successful, it must stick to its mission. . . . I hope that those who do not yet have an opinion about CFF will remain open-minded and recognize that its mission must be limited to research for success (participant 52, 1995)

There are other people living with CF who do not have strong opinions on these topics either way. The point to be made is simply that there is a diversity of opinion and there are people living with CF who are unhappy about the aggressive promotion of gene therapy research to the exclusion of many other, often more pressing, issues that make an impact on their lives.

Little systematic effort has been made to educate patients about gene therapy or to understand patients' feelings and concerns about gene therapy research in the larger context of their lives with CF. As the CFF sees 'the cure' for cystic fibrosis as its goal, it concentrates on research almost exclusively and, as a result, patient education and other support services have a low priority. Its fundraising activities are also fundamentally in conflict with patient education.

The CFF has, in fact, actively sought to isolate patients and family members from participating in discussion of clinical practice and research. For example, in 1996 non-professionals were refused admission to the NACF Conference, in striking contrast to CF conferences held in Canada and Europe, where lay participants have a recognised and visible presence. This became a topic of intense discussion on Cystic-L and in response a representative of the CFF's medical advisory committee (MAC), who had never previously posted a message and who was not known to be a subscriber by others on the list, posted the following ironic explanation:

All members of the MAC felt that open discussion—whose goal is to improve CF care and advance research—would be inhibited by lay attendance. MAC worries that conversation would be misinterpreted and false hopes, or worse, untrue failures, would be the message taken home: we don't need confusion/rumors about what is going on!

It may not be coincidental that at the previous conference there had been a public confrontation between one of the few adults with CF who had attended the conference and the CFF's president. The person in question had been openly critical of the CFF's financial practices and had set up an unofficial table to distribute a consumer newsletter.

The CFF has also been hostile to the activities of two former chapters in Florida and California that broke away in the 1970s and 1980s to establish independent organisations that were more responsive to the needs of local families living with CF. Both these groups, which have been financially successful, are closely allied with local CF centres, but in general independent groups find it difficult to sustain close co-operative relationships with clinicians and researchers. Only important CF centres with well-known researchers can afford or are willing to sustain this type of relationship in the face of pressure to stay strictly within the CFF's network of influence.

There is little evidence that bench scientists have any great interest in interacting with patients either, at least in the absence of an actual marketable product. Researchers rarely have to deal with patients as they consider that to be someone else's job. As one gene therapy researcher commented:

I don't think the patient enters our thinking as we try to develop intelligent systems and models and testing procedures. This is very much removed from the patient. . . . We don't really think of the patients. We leave that to the clinicians (interviewee 30, 1995).

When contact does occur, it occurs, according to the same interviewee, because it is initiated by patients:

Where it [the relationship with the patient] enters our thinking is when something becomes public information and is brought into the newspapers in a positive or negative fashion. In a positive fashion, you get immediate calls from all sorts of people who know your name through friends or just looked it up in the phone book or something: 'Well, can I come in and volunteer for this' (interviewee 30, 1995)?

Some gene researchers are both physicians and lab researchers but these individuals do not always meet patients either, even their research subjects. A South African, who was flown to New York to participate in a CF trial conducted by a well-known and much publicised gene therapy researcher, states of his experience: '. . . I professed interest to meet the trial leader, but over three visits he never took the trouble to meet with me' (Claassen 1998: 30). He goes on to recount the trouble he had getting any response from the research team after he returned to South Africa and contracted tuberculous, and of feeling that he was a 'guinea pig' who was 'expendable' after serving his purpose.

The relationship between physicians and researchers may be similarly distant. At the NACF conference and at other venues physicians are kept updated on progress in gene therapy research, which is usually the topic of one of the plenary talks, but there is relatively little interaction between the researchers and physicians at these conferences. Different professional groups often separate out into cliques that focus on their particular objects of professional interest: the pulmonary system, the gastrointestinal system, gene vectors, and so on (*cf.* Heath 1998). As one physician commented, '. . . not an awful lot of overlap. You go to the NACF meeting and nursing staff will be in forums with other nursing staff; gene therapy people will be with gene therapy people' (interviewee 29, 1995).

Physicians are the most sceptical group when it comes to gene therapy, although they do not generally voice their opinions publicly. Gene therapy is perceived as a potential treatment, but one that is unlikely to be available for years and which will probably be less than a cure. This understanding of gene therapy contrasts with the vision of gene therapy commonly broadcast by the biotechnology companies, the CFF, and the media. Physicians generally perceive scientific researchers and others as grossly underestimating, or at least downplaying, the clinical complexities of CF. As one physician observed derisively, 'Most bench scientists wouldn't know a CF patient if one came right up to them and coughed sputum' (interviewee 10, 1995). While attracted to the idea of modifying the basic mechanisms that cause the disease, physicians are less heavily invested in wonder drugs. Many of the older physicians have been listening to predictions of wonder drugs for decades, whereas the clinical reality for them has been one of slow and steady progress.

Physicians do not always convey their more sceptical attitude to their patients and their patients' families. Physicians, more than any other group, have to juggle many difficult and competing demands. In some situations it may be easier to put the best spin on a situation, although this is not always appreciated, as in this instance recounted by a mother of a young child with CF:

> . . . during this weak moment . . . I dared to utter that this disease is devastating, I received a CF pep talk from one of the docs. You know, the 'what a great time [in history] it is to have CF' talk. Sometimes, that just doesn't lessen the realities of the struggle we all face. . . . I, personally, need to know the present realities as well as the possibilities of a good future (participant 53, 1994)

There is also annoyance on the part of some that their physicians have not provided them with a realistic sense of the possibilities of gene therapy:

> . . . [one doctor] was giving very carefully filtered information—particularly about gene therapy, saying how well it's going—and I asked about the 'failure'—she redirected and gave a more truthful story. . . . I have come to accept it as a lecture type thing . . . there is no support (interviewee, 11, 1995).

These comments were made by a parent of a young boy with CF. Her comments refer to an exchange at a meeting held by her CF centre for patients and their families in late 1995. CF centres often hold such meetings immediately after the NACF Conference and are one of the main means through which centre staff communicate information about the latest research to patients. Adults with CF also express frustration with the lack of open communication about research, as in this instance:

> What has bothered me about clinicians is that when the super-hype about gene therapy was being spread around by the Foundation they didn't speak up. Many hide behind the mantle of 'not wanting to extinguish patients' hope', but fail to see how ungrounded this false hope is. It is the rare clinician who will speak openly to his patients about the promise of gene therapy. Without the help of knowledge and understanding from a clinician, patients have a difficult time weeding their way through the hype spread about by the Ron Crystals of the world (interviewee 23, 1996)

(Crystal was the first researcher to do CF gene therapy using human subjects and was a founder member of a biotechnology startup doing CF research in the early 1990s.)

While some physicians may merely lack the knowledge and skills necessary to discuss research effectively with their patients, there are other factors complicating the doctor–patient relationship. Physicians at the specialist centres, where most CF patients receive their care, may have numerous reasons for not voicing critical opinions on gene therapy research. Many of these centres have been under considerable financial and institutional pressures in recent years and need to maintain good relationships with researchers and the support of the CFF. Income from a large clinical trial can pay a significant part of the salary of a clinical co-ordinator or another team member. Physicians are sometimes quite explicit about this, as in the case of the following CF centre director whose centre was about to undertake a large CF gene therapy study:

> One of the major reasons for doing drug studies—aside from the possible efficacy of the agent—is money. A lot of these trials are done now by pharmaceutical companies and for the study they do allow you a certain amount of funding per patient enrollment. . . . We were like many institutions also attracted by the monies because we need monies to fund people . . . [from the amiloride study] we got funding for a nurse, a full-time nurse, which helps the functioning of the clinic (interviewee 16, 1994)

For most physicians, given the small and tightly organised professional relationships surrounding CF, there is little to be gained by being openly critical of research publicity, and there are often too many pressures on their time to allow them to mediate research publicity effectively for their patients.

These issues aside, there is almost no research addressing the concern that Orkin and Motulusky (1995) raise that patients and parents may make unwise decisions based on the publicity surrounding gene therapy research. Decisions might include joining a waiting list for lung transplantation or reproductive choices. There is evidence to suggest that some adults with CF do not understand the different forms gene therapy research can take and the limitations of those forms. It is not clear that most patients appreciate the difference between the insertion of a gene into a lung epithelial cell and gene repair, or that CF gene therapy will not repair damaged lung tissue. An adult man with CF, for example, made the following comment to Cystic-L in 1998:

> My understanding of these ongoing gene therapy trials, is that healthy genes are inserted into lung tissue DNA through some vector with the hope that these cells will reproduce and eventually give you a new set of CF-free lungs (participant 54, 1998).

In a study of patients enrolled in a phase I trial in the United Kingdom, the researchers noted that most patients had an 'emotionally driven optimism about gene therapy', and a preference for the potential of gene therapy over heart-lung transplantation (Blair *et al.* 1998, 218), although it is not clear what bearing this preference might have on clinical decisions.

**Conclusion**

At the moment it is not clear what sort of benefits gene therapy research will eventually bring to people with diseases like CF. Given time, gene therapy may yet prove to be a revolutionary medical technology. Regardless of what is eventually accomplished, the issue raised here concerns the nature of the research process and its consequences for people with CF. The process has reduced the desires and needs of people with CF to a cure at all costs. This suggests a lack of understanding for the many ways people live with and experience the disease.

The CFF's choice to focus on research for a 'cure' has meant that the many other potentially competing needs of people with CF and their families, such as CF education, social support, and age-appropriate care, have been marginalised. This has ensured that a concentrated and extremely successful research strategy is not diluted. The CFF has been able to accomplish this because it has established itself at the centre of a powerful network of clinical and well-funded research centres.

Despite claims to the contrary, consumers are often in a weak position to play an active role in biomedical research. Patients and their families who are not in accord with the CFF's narrow research agenda are not in a position to impose an alternative agenda. They constitute a relatively small group, around 20,000 to 25,000 in the United states, are dispersed, and have no common bond to unite around other than CF. This makes them unlike the few consumer groups, such as AIDS activist groups, whose size, concentration and existing political structures have enabled them to exploit the media, professional differences and their role as human research subjects, to obtain a significant role in shaping the research process (Epstein 1995).

There are important differences of opinion between clinicians and researchers, and even amongst gene therapy researchers, on the nature of the process of CF gene therapy research. Clinicians in particular are likely to be more sceptical of gene therapy research and are in a position to convey a more critical perspective to their patients. However, resource pressures on CF centres, the relatively weak position of clinical interests relative to research interests and the close-knit relationships surrounding CF research and care have meant that there is little opportunity or incentive for clinicians to voice their differences publicly or more effectively to mediate the publicity surrounding gene therapy research for the benefit of their patients.

## Acknowledgements

The author wishes to acknowledge comments from the editors and the anonymous referees who commented on earlier versions of this chapter.

## References

Anonymous (1993) Advertising by medical charities (Editorial), *Lancet*, 342, 1187–8.

Bayertz, K., Paslack, R. and Schmidt, K.W. (1994) Summary of 'gene transfer into human somatic cells. State of the technology, medical risks, social and ethical problems: a report', *Human Gene Therapy*, 5, 465–8.

Blair, C., Kacser, E. and Porteous, D. (1998) Gene therapy for cystic fibrosis: a psychosocial study of trial participants, *Gene Therapy*, 5, 218–22.

Brown, K. (1996) Industry researchers decry tone of NIH gene therapy report, *The Scientist*, 19 February.

Claassen, C. (1998) A personal account of a gene therapy trial, *IACFA Newsletter*, August.

Cystic Fibrosis Foundation (1997) *Patient Registry 1996 Annual Data Report*. Bethesda, MD: Cystic Fibrosis Foundation.

Durant, J., Hansen, A. and Bauer, M. (1996) Public understanding of the new genetics. In Marteau, T. and Richards, M. (eds) *The Troubled Helix: Social and Psychological Implications of the New Human Genetics*. Cambridge: Cambridge University Press.

Epstein, S. (1995) The construction of lay expertise: AIDS activism and the forging of credibility in the reform of clinical trials, *Science, Technology and Human Values*, 20, 408–37.

Fletcher, J.C. (1990) Evolution of ethical debate about human gene therapy, *Human Gene Therapy*, 1, 55–68.

Friedmann, T. (1996) Human gene therapy—an immature genie, but certainly out of the bottle, *Nature Medicine*, 2, 144–7.

Gorman, C. (1995) Has gene therapy stalled? *Time Magazine*, 9 October.

Gustavson, J. (1997) An insider's view of gene therapy, *Bay Area Reporter*, 24 April.

Hahn, R.A. and Kleinman, A. (1983) Biomedical practice and anthropological theory, *Annual Review of Anthropology*, 12, 305–33.

Hannerz, U. (1992) *Cultural Complexity: Studies in the Social Organization of Meaning*. New York: Columbia University Press.

Heath, D. (1998) Locating genetic knowledge: picturing marfan syndrome and traveling constituencies. *Science, Technology and Human Values*, 23, 71–97.

Hillman, A.L., Brenner, M.K., Caplan, A.L., Carey, J., Champey, Y., Culver, K.W., Drummond, M.F., Freund, D.A., Holmes, E.W., Kelley, W.N., Kolata, G., Levine, M.N., Levy, E., Schondelmeyer, S.W., Velu, T. and Wilson, J.M. (1996) Gene therapy: socioeconomic and ethical issues. A roundtable discussion, *Human Gene Therapy*, 7, 1139–44.

Hofman, K.J., Tambor, E.S., Chase, G.A., Geller, G., Faden, R.R. and Holtzman, N.A. (1993) Physicians' knowledge of genetics and genetic tests, *Academic Medicine*, 68, 625–32.

Kerr, A., Cunningham-Burley, S. and Amos, A. (1997) The new genetics: professionals' discursive boundaries, *The Sociological Review*, 45, 280–303.

Kerr, A., Cunningham-Burley, S. and Amos, A. (1998) Drawing the line: an analysis of lay people's discussions about the new genetics, *Public Understanding of Science*, 7, 113–33.

Marcus, G.E. (1995) Ethnography in/of the world system: the emergence of multi-sited ethnography, *Annual Review of Anthropology*, 24, 95–117.

Martin, P. and Thomas, S.M. (1996) *The Development of Gene Therapy in Europe and the United States: a Comparative Analysis*. Brighton: Science Policy Research Unit, Sussex University.

Maugh, T. (1990) Gene therapy offers hope for cystic fibrosis, *Los Angeles Times*, 21 September.

Maugh, T. (1992) Cystic fibrosis: cure seen in gene therapy, *Los Angeles Times*, 10 January.

Mulligan, R.C. (1993) The basic science of gene therapy, *Science*, 260, 926–32.

Murray, T.H. (1990) Human gene therapy, the public, and public policy, *Human Gene Therapy*, 1, 49–54.

Office of Inspector General (1998) *Institutional Review Boards: a Time for Reform*. Washington, D.C.: Government Printing Office.

Orkin, S.H. and Motulsky, A.G. (1995) *Report and Recommendations of The Panel to Assess the NIH Investment in Research on Gene Therapy*, (http://www.nih. gov/news/panelrep.html). Bethesda, MD: National Institutes of Health.

Palca, J. (1995) Gene therapy produces disappointing results, *All Things Considered*, National Public Radio, 27 September.

Purvis, A. (1992) Laying siege to a deadly gene, *Time Magazine*, 24 February.

Recombinant DNA Advisory Committee (1994) *Minutes of Meeting, 12–13 September, 1998*. Bethesda, MD: National Institutes of Health.

Rensberger, B. (1992) New therapy is major step to a 'cure' for cystic fibrosis, *Philadelphia Inquirer*, 10 January.

Richards, M. (1996) Lay and professional knowledge of genetics and inheritance, *Public Understanding of Science*, 5, 217–30.

Southwick, K. (1995) Plying a murky gene-therapy pool; biotechnology: a promising field is hindered by red tape, money problems and greed, *Los Angeles Times*, 22 March.

Turney, J. (1995) The public understanding of genetics—where next? *European Journal of Genetics and Society*, 1, 5–20.

Walters, L. (1991) Human gene therapy: ethics and public policy, *Human Gene Therapy*, 2, 115–22.

Young, A. (1982) The anthropologies of illness and sickness, *Annual Review of Anthropology*, 11, 257–85.

Zallen, D.T. (1996) Public oversight is necessary if human gene therapy is to progress, *Human Gene Therapy*, 7, 795–7.

# Doing the right thing: genetic risk and responsibility

*Nina Hallowell*

## Introduction

The cloning of genes which predispose individuals to inherited disorders (for example, cystic fibrosis), and the reclassification of common diseases (for example, breast cancer) as having a genetic origin in a subset of cases, coupled with the advent of predictive genetic testing, are presented as providing individuals with new choices for managing their health. The rhetoric of the new genetics claims the knowledge provided as a result of genetic testing is empowering (Petersen 1998). However, in practice, it has been observed that individuals who undergo genetic testing often perceive their freedom to choose between the different options on offer as constrained in a variety of ways, for example, by personal circumstances or the context of test provision. In particular, they frequently report feeling that their choice of 'not knowing' is limited (Kerr and Cunningham-Burley 1998). Similarly, Katz Rothman (1994) observes that the choices available to women following an amniocentesis are so constrained that those who test positive do not experience themselves as choosing between the limited options, but as being trapped by this knowledge and the responsibility it entails.

This chapter demonstrates that the choices available to women who are identified as (potentially) at genetic risk of developing breast/ovarian cancer are similarly constrained. It will argue that one of the constraints on women's choices derives from their perception that they have a responsibility to other people not only to determine their risks, but also to take steps to control them in some way.

## Health risks and responsibility

The idea that individuals should take responsibility for their health is implicitly assumed by most health promotion campaigns (Baric 1969, Crawford 1977, Graham 1979, Lupton 1993, 1995, Petersen and Lupton 1996) and also invoked in lay accounts of health behaviour (Backett 1992, Pill and Stott 1982). For example, Backett (1992) reports that middle class family members consider it important to present an image of behaving responsibly with regard to their own health and the health of their children. Similarly, a study of lay explanations of the aetiology of illness found that although the majority of the participants regarded illness as having external causes, many accepted a limited degree of responsibility for their health, insofar as they acknowledged that their behaviour may compromise their inbuilt resistance to disease (Pill and Stott 1982).

Individuals are not only encouraged to take responsibility for their own health, but also the health of others. For example, the basic premise of HIV/AIDS awareness campaigns is that individuals have a responsibility to indulge in 'good' or 'approved' sexual practices to protect themselves *and* their sexual partners from exposure to the risk of infection (Odets 1995, Patton 1993). Lay accounts suggest that individuals readily accept responsibility for others' health. For example, Graham (1979) observes that mothers not only assume the responsibility for maintaining and promoting their children's health, but frequently place the family's health needs above their own. Similarly, Howson argues that women perceive themselves as behaving responsibly by undergoing cervical screening, and regard themselves as having an obligation 'to inform and persuade friends and kin of the necessity of [cervical] screening' (1998: 230).

The construction of health as a moral issue has generally been confined to discussions of voluntary health risks—people's lifestyle choices or behaviour. More recently it has been observed that individuals not only have a responsibility to avoid voluntarily exposing themselves and others to health risks, but also may be seen as bearing some responsibility for their genetic risks (Kenen 1994, Lupton 1995, Steinberg 1996, Tong 1997, Petersen 1998).

Biomedical discourses construct genetic risks as internally imposed involuntary health risks. However, the fact that these risks are involuntary does not absolve gene carriers of responsibility for their health. Indeed, it can be argued that because genetic risks are portrayed as part of the individual's make up their responsibility to act to protect their health, or the health of future generations, is emphasised, for inherited risk can not be blamed upon external sources.[1] This responsibility is accentuated within genetic consultations which not only identify the precise risks to an individual's health (or the health of their offspring) but, by promoting self-surveillance, also promise individuals control over these uncertainties (Castel 1991, Petersen 1998). Indeed, it can be argued that by labelling individuals as 'at-risk', and presenting genetic risks as manageable, genetic counselling implicitly places individuals under an obligation to attempt to modify these risks.

The new genetics not only positions individuals as responsible for their own health, but also for the health of others. Steinberg argues that women, in particular, have come to be seen as bearing the responsibility for genetic risks. She observes that genetic discourses construct women as 'the bearers of "nature's defects"' or 'gene transmitters' (1996: 267) and as such, they are seen as, almost single-handedly, bearing the responsibility for passing on their own *and* their partner's genes. She argues that genetic screening presents women with a paradox, if they choose to undertake screening in order to avoid the 'disempowering and often punitive social consequences of bearing and caring for a disabled child' (1996: 267), then they implicitly reinforce those (obstetric and eugenic) discourses which can be seen as a source of disempowerment.

Similarly, Kenen (1994) speculates about the extent to which the new genetics has the potential to alter our notions of responsibility for the health of others. She observes that advances in genetic technologies may fundamentally alter the way we view the self, in relation to others. She argues that the increasing availability of genetic information may result in individuals developing a sense of 'genetic responsibility'—an obligation to reveal genetic information about the self to their kin. She observes that this in turn may lead to a shift away from the western view of the autonomous or independent self to a more 'interdependent' self (1994: 57), in which the needs of significant others are seen as an integral part of the self.

In summary, the existing literature suggests that individuals not only assume the responsibility for maintaining their own health, but also the health of others. This chapter addresses the question of whether individuals similarly regard themselves as having a responsibility for their genetic risks. Using data collected during a prospective study of women attending genetic counselling for hereditary breast/ovarian cancer (HBOC) it will demonstrate that women who are identified as at-risk not only assume responsibility for their own and others' genetic risks, but also perceive themselves as having an obligation to others to manage these risks. It will be argued that by constructing genetic risk and risk management as a moral issue these women relinquish their right to not know about their genetic risk and constrain their risk management choices.

It is important first to outline the choices that are available to women who have a family history of breast/ovarian cancer. The next section will provide a brief review of the risks of developing cancer and the costs and benefits of the risk management options.

## Hereditary breast/ovarian cancer: what are the risks and risk management options?

Between five–10 per cent of cases of breast and ovarian cancer are caused by an inherited predisposition. Some of the genes responsible for causing these cancers have recently been identified (Miki et al. 1994, Wooster et al. 1994). It is calculated that mutation carriers have a breast cancer risk which may be as high as 85 per cent and an ovarian cancer risk which may be as high as 60 per cent (Easton et al. 1995, Tonin et al. 1995). Women who have a family history of these cancers are referred for genetic counselling, where their risks of carrying a mutation and developing cancer are calculated, and different risk management options are discussed.

At the present time the identification of a woman's genetic risk status is usually based upon the type of family history she presents (i.e. the number, type and ages of affected relatives). Although genetic screening is available, the practice is not widespread. Technically this is a difficult procedure and therefore, DNA-testing is normally confined to women from multi-case families once the mutation has been identified in affected relatives. However, despite the fact that only a few women receive genetic confirmation of their risk status, many more are identified as being 'at risk' because of their family history. All at-risk women, i.e. confirmed and potential mutation carriers, are encouraged to adopt cancer risk management practices.

The first option offered to (potential) mutation carriers is annual screening, i.e. mammography plus clinical breast examination or ovarian ultrasound plus CA125 serum estimation (N.I.H. 1994). The rationale for screening is that cancers may be identified at an early stage when the prognosis is good. However, there are no data to indicate that breast/ovarian screening is effective in reducing mortality in high risk groups (Neugut and Jacobson 1995). Moreover, there is evidence that screening carries risks. First, interval cancers may occur or tumours may be missed altogether. Indeed, it is widely accepted that mammography is less effective in detecting cancers in younger women because of the density of the breast tissue. Second, screening may have iatrogenic consequences. The rate of false positives is significant,[2] and this may result in women having unnecessary exploratory operations. In addition, it has been calculated that annual exposure to radiation may compound the risk of developing breast cancer in gene carriers (Den Otter et al. 1996).

Alternatively, (potential) gene carriers can decrease their risk by undergoing prophylactic surgery—bilateral oophorectomy or mastectomy. A recent study suggests that prophylactic mastectomy confers a 90 per cent reduction in breast cancer risk (Hartmann et al. 1997). However, there is no evidence to indicate a reduction in mortality following prophylactic oophorectomy. Indeed, breast and 'extra-ovarian' tumours have been documented as occurring following prophylactic surgery (Ziegler and Kroll 1991, Stephanek et al. 1995 Tobacman et al. 1982, Piver et al. 1993). Furthermore, it is unclear whether the potential reduction in cancer risk following oophorectomy outweighs the risks of surgical menopause—the increased risks of cardiovascular disease, osteoporosis and other menopausal symptoms (Burke et al. 1997).[3] In the case of women who opt for breast reconstruction following prophylactic mastectomy there is ongoing debate about the risks of connective tissue disease associated with silicon breast implants (Cooper and Dennison 1998). Finally, surgery itself carries risks, those, for example, associated with anaesthesia and post-operative complications such as infections.

In addition to the medical risks, it must be noted that cancer risk management may have psychosocial repercussions. Research suggests that breast/ovarian screening may increase anxiety in high-risk women (Kash et al. 1992, Lerman and Schwartz 1993, Wardle 1995). Although there is evidence that women who undergo prophylactic surgery experience a decrease in cancer worries (Pernet *et al.* 1992, Stephanek *et al.* 1995), other research indicates that some women perceive their gender identity as compromised following prophylactic mastectomy (Hallowell 1999) and their lives as negatively affected by the menopausal symptoms they experience following prophylactic oophorectomy (Hallowell, 1998b). One of the problems with these studies is that little is known of the long-term consequences of this type of surgery.

Finally, it must be noted that although at-risk women can opt for no further medical intervention following their attendance at genetic counselling, this option is not included in the recommended guidelines for managing high-risk women (N.I.H. 1994). Observations of genetic consultations indicate that although the costs and benefits of screening/surgery are routinely described, the option of no further intervention is rarely mentioned, or is dismissed as inappropriate (Hallowell, 1998a).

Despite the fact that only a small proportion of women are thought to carry genetic mutations which predispose them to develop these cancers, the geneticisation (Lippman 1992) of breast/ovarian cancer has led to the recategorisation of many healthy women (and their offspring) as potentially 'at-risk'. This may not only have implications for one's identity, but also, as the above discussion suggests, one's health and emotional wellbeing; for the geneticisation of breast/ovarian cancer has meant that many healthy women have adopted risk management practices which may have iatrogenic consequences. The question this chapter addresses is what motivates healthy women to expose themselves to the risks associated with these risk management practices?

## The present study

### Recruitment
The participants were recruited from the Cambridge Family History clinic, where they had been referred for genetic counselling for HBOC. Excluding those who had had cancer, or had previously had genetic counselling, all women attending the clinic between February 1994 and February 1995 were invited to participate. Fifty-nine eligible women were approached, five did not reply and eight refused. Reasons for refusal included a reluctance to have a researcher present during the consultation or an unwillingness to have their consultation/interviews tape-recorded. Forty-six women were recruited.

### Data collection
All genetic consultations were observed (n = 46). In-depth interviews (n = 40) took place within two months of the consultation. One woman declined to be interviewed post-clinic and an interview was deemed inappropriate in five cases, for example, because of a recent bereavement. The

women were informed that the interviews would focus upon their: family history of cancer, experiences of genetic counselling, risk management decisions and general health behaviour. At the start of the interview the participants were asked to provide a narrative account of their experiences of the cancers in their family and what they had done since they became aware that they might be at-risk. Although the structure and content of the interview was dictated by the participants' initial responses, a series of probes, based upon the aforementioned themes, was used to guide the interviews.

With the exception of five women who had moved without leaving a forwarding address, all the interviewees were contacted a year later by telephone. These semi-structured interviews (n = 35) focused on risk management during the interim period and satisfaction with genetic counselling. The interviews were carried out by the author and two co-workers (H. Statham and F. Murton), the participants were interviewed by the same interviewer on both occasions. All interviews and consultations were tape-recorded with consent and transcribed. This chapter primarily uses data obtained during the in-depth interviews.

*Data analysis*
A thematic analysis of the consultations and interviews was carried out. The transcripts were initially coded according to categories based upon the interview themes, and emerging themes within the data were then identified and subsequently refined. Atlas-ti (Muhr 1994), a qualitative data analysis software package, was used to manage the data.

*Sample characteristics*
*Cancer family history* Eight women had a family history of breast and ovarian cancer, 18 breast cancer only, 12 ovarian cancer only and two a family history of breast and uterine/stomach cancer. A total of 123 relatives were reported as affected by breast/ovarian cancer (mean 3, range 1–8) and a further 66 male and female relatives as affected by other cancers. 98 per cent of the participants had a first degree relative affected by breast/ovarian cancer (Table 1). Nine women reported breast/ovarian cancer in one generation, 26 in two, four in three and one in four generations. Four women reported breast/ovarian cancer in paternal relatives, in one of these cases the cancers were confined to the paternal line.

*Mode of referral* The participants were referred to the clinic by either a general practitioner, gynaecologist or breast specialist. Data on referral patterns is available for 30 participants. The majority of participants had initiated the referral: six women reported that they had specifically asked for a referral to genetic counselling, 17 said they had asked their general practitioner for something to be done about the history of cancer in their family, in most cases this was an enquiry about the possibility of breast/ovarian screening, and the remaining seven women were identified as needing a referral by a medical practitioner.

Table 1:  *Percentage of women reporting relatives affected with breast or ovarian cancer*

|  |  | n | % |
|---|---|---|---|
| First generation | Mother | 26 | 65 |
|  | Sister | 13 | 33 |
|  |  | 39 |  |
| Second generation | Paternal half-sister | 1 | 3 |
|  | Maternal Aunt | 17 | 43 |
|  | Paternal Aunt | 2 | 5 |
|  | Maternal Grandmother | 16 | 40 |
|  | Paternal Grandmother | 2 | 5 |
|  |  | 38 |  |
| Third generation | Maternal Cousin | 8 | 20 |
|  | Paternal Cousin | 1 | 3 |
|  | Maternal Great Grandmother | 2 | 5 |
|  | Maternal Great Aunt | 2 | 5 |
|  |  | 13 |  |
| Fourth generation | Maternal Second Cousin | 1 | 3 |
|  | Paternal Second Cousin | 1 | 3 |
|  |  | 2 |  |

*Demographic characteristics*  Thirty-six women were married/living as married, three were divorced/separated and one was single. Thirty-two women had children, 28 at least one daughter and 25 at least one son. One woman was pregnant with her first child. Twenty women had completed their education at 16 years, seven at 18 years and 11 had received education beyond the age of 18. Occupational (Table 2) and employment data were available for 39 women. Twenty-nine women were in paid employment, (12 full-time, 17 part-time) and two were full-time students in higher education. Seven women had worked at some time in a job with a medical connection (for example, doctor, nurse or receptionist in a medical practice).

### Discussions of risk management during genetic counselling

The clinic was run by two oncologists (one male, one female) working in the field of cancer genetics research. In every session the clinician estimated the woman's risk and discussed the risk management options. The risks of carrying a mutation and developing cancer were calculated purely on the basis of the family history presented. The clinicians stressed that the probabilities they provided were estimates, and that risk could only be predicted more accurately if, and when, a woman's carrier status was established either by mutation testing or by confirmation of their family history. Predictive

Table 2: *Participants' occupational background*

| Professional Groupings* | (n=35) | % |
|---|---|---|
| Managers and Administrators | 3 | 9 |
| Professional | 5 | 14 |
| Associate Professional and Technical | 6 | 17 |
| Clerical and Secretarial | 11 | 31 |
| Craft and Related | 1 | 3 |
| Personal and Protective Service | 6 | 17 |
| Sales | 0 | 0 |
| Plant and Machine Operatives | 2 | 6 |
| Others | 1 | 3 |

* OPCS 1992 Census

testing was not offered to any of the participants during this study. Given the incomplete penetrance of the genes which predispose individuals to develop these cancers and the fact that none of the women had genetic confirmation of their carrier status, the highest numerical risk estimate for developing cancer given to a woman in this study was 40 per cent, the lowest three per cent.

Three courses of action were discussed during the consultations: breast and/or ovarian screening (all consultations), prophylactic surgery (28 sessions), and the option of no further intervention generally described by the clinicians as 'doing nothing' (nine sessions). As I have discussed elsewhere (Hallowell 1998a), although the clinicians stressed that their recommendations were dependent upon confirmation of risk status, by framing the different risk management options in different ways, they can be seen as implicitly encouraging these women to engage in particular types of risk management behaviour. Thus, some options—breast/ovarian screening and prophylactic oophorectomy—were presented as not only appropriate but 'responsible' behaviour, while others—no medical intervention or prophylactic mastectomy—were either not discussed or dismissed as inappropriate.

### Women's perceptions of risk

Throughout the interviews, cancer was described as a silent and deadly disease. It was seen as the danger within—'the silent killer' that strikes without warning, and 'eats away at your body'. It was regarded as unpredictable insofar as one could not know when it would strike, but predictable to the extent that most women thought that it would strike them at some time. As one woman said: 'I've always felt it was like a finger pointing at me, you know, like a Monty Python-like finger'.

Despite the fact that one of the aims of genetic counselling is to quantify uncertainty by providing counsellees with a probabilistic analysis of their risks, many of these women described their risk in absolute rather than probabilistic terms—they felt they would definitely develop cancer in the future. The probabilities discussed during genetic counselling did not appear to change their beliefs, as one woman said:

> . . . She explained it very well, you know, she said, one in eleven women will get it during their lifetime you're sort of one in five, because you're higher. . . . It doesn't sound that horrific. . . . I wanted to hear that, but I still thought, well, I'm still going to get it. Because that's the way I am. . . . I've said straight from the start, it's too close to me for me to just brush it off (P11).

The fact that these women tended not to perceive their risk as a neutral probability is not surprising, for it is generally accepted that lay perceptions of risk are value-laden (Douglas and Wildavsky 1982, Douglas 1990). There is evidence that many individuals who attend genetic counselling convert the risk estimations they receive into binary terms, i.e. X either will or will not occur (Lippman-Hand and Fraser 1979a, 1979b, Parsons and Atkinson 1992, Parsons and Clarke 1993), and that risk perception is influenced by personal and social factors (Pearn 1973). Similar observations were made in this study which indicated that in many cases risk perception was influenced by the experience of cancer in the family—particularly witnessing the death of close relatives. As one woman said: 'When my mum was really unwell I definitely was depressed and said "well I am definitely going to get cancer I should think", it was very awesome. No two ways about it' (GC22). Other factors affecting risk perception, included: lay theories about the aetiology of cancer, the influence, for example, of personality factors, stress and environmental 'triggers', beliefs about their health, particularly the ability of their body to ward off the effects of stress and environmental toxins, and their understanding of genetics. In many cases risk perception was influenced by a combination of these. One woman, for example, subscribed to the theory that cancer was caused by the interaction of stressful events with certain personality types. She reasoned that she would inevitably develop cancer because she had inherited personality traits from her mother which made her susceptible to the negative effects of stress.

## Women's perceptions of responsibility

Although many women regarded cancer as a predictable outcome, given their family history, all saw themselves as having a responsibility to act to avert this danger if possible. Their attendance at generic counselling was perceived as the first step in taking responsibility for their risks, and was influenced by obligations to their kin. The importance of putting others' needs before their own was stressed throughout the interviews, and their (intended) actions were justified almost exclusively in terms of the implications for other people. All the women described their attendance at genetic counselling as being of direct benefit to their family or researchers. They said they had a responsibility to past, present and future generations to *determine* and *manage* their risks.

*Responsibility to determine risk*

> ... maybe if they find out that I do have this gene ... I can be more honest with myself and honest with the family, you know, my family (GC22)

Genetics is not about individuals, it is about biological relationships. One's genetic risk is, by definition, shared with other biological relatives. Therefore, to have genetic information about oneself, is to have information about others. This observation has lead Kenen (1994) to speculate that one of the consequences of the geneticisation of life may be a shift in how one thinks of oneself in relation to others. She predicts that the increasing focus on biological connections may have social consequences, in the sense that it may result in individuals developing a sense of 'genetic responsibility' towards others.

The idea that individuals are not only responsible for their own risks, but also those of other family members' (children, sisters, nieces, cousins, aunts and mothers) was frequently expressed. During genetic counselling these women not only found out about their own risks, but also learned of other family members' risks. Many women described themselves as not only having a responsibility to inform their relatives of these risks, but also talked about their relatives' right to have the information they had obtained.

> I do keep other family members informed of what goes on. When I came back from the clinic I said to [sister], you know, this is what they said, they think that you should be in a screening programme just like me. So go to the doctor and do something about it. As of yet she hasn't gone to the doctor and done anything about it. I can only tell her. What she does with that information I give her is up to her, as with other members of my family. I can only share the information that I get (P11).

All had discussed the content of the counselling session with at least one biological relative by the time of the interview, and most intended to contact other relatives to give them this information. Some women acknowledged that this might be difficult because they did not know these relatives, their relatives had been recently bereaved or were estranged from the family. However, the women said they had a duty to disseminate this information within their family, no matter how difficult that might be. Indeed, their feelings of genetic responsibility meant that many women were prepared to compromise other family members' rights of 'not knowing' about their genetic status, for example:

> . . . this daughter that I had adopted I wouldn't generally contact at all because I don't even know if she knows she's adopted . . . But if I'd been told there was a very great risk, and if I happen to get it, I would find some way of passing the information on, because I would feel that's a moral duty really (GC12).

However, most were concerned that the disclosure of genetic information might provoke anxiety in more vulnerable family members (the young, the ill and the aged), and some went to great lengths to shield them from this information.

Some women not only felt they had an obligation to provide their kin with information about risk and risk management, but also said they had a responsibility to persuade their relatives to act upon this information. Indeed, one woman, who had no children of her own, admitted using emotional blackmail to convince her sister to take up breast screening:

> I mean I'm not on a crusade to get everyone going [to screening], but I would like to think that they [family] thought it as important an issue as I do, especially [sister]. I mean I really do want her to go, and I've tried the tack, 'well, you've got daughters now so you've really got to start thinking of them' (P11).

Miller (1976) argues that serving the needs of others is so important to a woman's sense of identity, that others' needs come to be identified as her own. In other words, women's actions are guided by others' needs. Likewise, many of the women in the present study said they had come to counselling because they needed to determine the potential risks to other family members, and to establish what they could do about risk management. Many women acknowledged that they felt responsible for having put their children at risk.[5] As one woman said:

> Because I mean a large—with hindsight, a large proportion of my concern was a responsibility to my daughter. And I think also it's sort of helplessness. You know? I've passed on the gene to my daughter. I must make sure that I, you know, alert her to the possibilities, because I mean it's not fault but it's a kind of responsibility (GC13).

Some of those who did not have children expressed similar sentiments. They said it was important to determine one's risk status so that one could obtain information for future children or other relatives, such as siblings. Indeed, nearly all the women regarded the provision of information about the risk status of other relatives, particularly children and sisters, as one of the most important benefits of DNA-testing.[6]

But even though you know that you've got the gene, it's not very easy to sort of say how you are going to feel until you actually find out you have got it. But also it's handy to know if I had a daughter. So that's how I feel really, you know, for my family really. Because you feel—I mean you have all these maybe hereditary illnesses that you think, should I have children, should I not? And if you're passing something on down to your child, you obviously want to know the best way of coping with it and then letting them know what's happening, you know, you've got to be open with them, otherwise problems occur (GC22).

Some women said that if they were offered a predictive test in the future, then they would take it purely for this reason. As one woman who had no children said:

Well, it's easy to say I'd want it but don't know what benefits I'd get from it. But I just want to know if I'd inherited it. And then know if I would give it to my children or if I didn't have it then there wouldn't be the faulty gene to pass down (GC35).

Even those who acknowledged that having a positive test result would cause them anxiety or might have negative implications for their employment and insurance, said they would be prepared to undergo testing because they had a responsibility to provide others with this information.

I'd be frightened to have it but I think I would have it. I would have it because I think it would be something I would regret later on, . . . And also I think it would be only right for me to have it because I've got three daughters. I think I would owe it to them to have it done as well (GC04).

Thus, for many of these women their feelings of genetic responsibility meant that they were prepared to compromise their own needs of 'not knowing' their risks for the sake of others. One woman described how her husband had used the argument that she had a responsibility to their children to get her to confront her fears about finding out about her risk status:

And I just said to him [husband], I don't want to know. If I'm going to get it [cancer], then I just want to get it. I don't want to go for this test. And he kept saying, well you know, you should, because not just for you, but for the kids, and everything like that. And I said, I don't care, whatever's going to be is going to be (GC25).

Finally, the women talked about the need to obtain knowledge for future generations. Only two women said the information they received during counselling might have influenced their earlier reproductive decisions. Both felt that it was important for their children to have this information so that they could make informed reproductive decisions in the future.

Um . . . well, I know what my chances are of getting it [gene], and if I get it then I'll deal with it, you know. I think it would be nice for her [daughter] to know whether she has got it or hasn't got it, so she's got a choice whether she wants to have children or not. I mean I didn't realise, or I might have thought again about having children if I'd have realised that, you know, I could pass on a defunct gene. I might have adopted instead of having my own children, after seeing my mother die and what my sister's been through (GC17).

Many women also talked about their responsibilities to ensure the wellbeing of women in general. They said they felt that they had an obligation to contribute to research on the genetics of breast/ovarian cancer for the benefit of future generations, and expressed the hope that the information they provided about their family would advance knowledge.[7]

. . . and the fact that I've got information to give, and I want to pass it on, and I want to pass it on to anybody else that could benefit from it. If, through our family it isolates another chain, then that's wonderful. I mean it's something. But I think any information. I know genes are something you've got and you can't alter, but I think if you have something in you, you can use that; I think if you have something that is benefiting research, I don't think you have the right to withhold it . . . (GC37).

To summarise, throughout these accounts the self was not presented as an individuated or autonomous agent, but repeatedly constructed in-relation to others (Gilligan 1982)—as an 'interdependent' self (Kenen 1994). Although all these women had already identified themselves as at-risk before they attended this clinic, they described their motivations to determine the extent of their risk as influenced by others' needs for information. Genetic information was perceived as information about 'the family' and as such, they reasoned that they had an obligation to ensure that all their kin had access to this information. In some cases their own needs of not knowing about their risk status were regarded as subordinate to what they perceived as others' needs. Thus, it could be argued that the feelings of genetic responsibility expressed by these women ultimately threatened their autonomy, insofar as they constrained their choices, particularly their right not to know about their genetic risks.

*Obligations to manage risk*
There was evidence that these women not only saw themselves as connected to others in a biological sense but perceived themselves as an integral part of a complex web of social relationships which carried with it a set of obligations of care (Mason 1996). These obligations were described as influencing their cancer risk management decisions.

Nine women had been alerted by a dying relative (mother, sister or cousin) to the possibility that cancer might be inherited in their family. She had insisted that they seek advice about their risks and do something to protect themselves. They recognised that their relative had been motivated by feelings of responsibility towards them.

> It was last year mum did say to me, you've got to make sure that everything is all right. And I think in a way at the back of her mind she felt guilty because, you know, you're not very well and you think about your child, that it could happen to them, the same way as I would feel that, you know, there's not much you can do but tell them how you feel (GC22).

All these women said they had felt under an obligation to fulfil the undertaking they had made to their dying relatives to determine and manage their risk. One woman described how her feelings of responsibility to her mother had helped her to overcome her fear of going to the clinic:

> . . . and my mother came over to see me just before she died and she knew she was dying, I knew she was dying, . . . and the last thing she said to me was, look your great-grannie's dead, your grandmother's dead, your sister's dead, and I'm next on the list . . . Now is the time to start making some decisions. And I promised my mother, the last thing she said to me was, if there's ever anything that you can do, genetic testing, blood tests, and she promised, she said, I'll haunt you if you don't go and get your smears regularly, I will haunt you. And that was the reason why I got in touch with my doctor, and that was the reason why I decided to have the genetic counselling. If it minimises my risk, then that was the one thing I was going to have, and that's why I had it done . . . and it took a lot of courage (GC01).

More frequently, women described their risk management decisions as influenced by their obligations to living relatives. Many said that it was not until they had the responsibility of caring for children that they had started to worry about their risk.

> Yes, I think it was then that I started to think, oh, perhaps—and you see when my mother died I hadn't got children of my own, and I don't—I think, you know, I have responsibilities now, and it makes you think more about your health, doesn't it, because you think, if anything happens, what's going to happen to my children? And that's my biggest concern, is my children. I mean I don't want to die of cancer, obviously, but my concern didn't come until after my children, really, I think anyway (GC10).

All those who had children, said that their intention to undertake some form of risk management stemmed from a feeling of duty to their children.

They described themselves as having a responsibility to remain healthy so that they were able to engage in the practice of 'mothering work' *i.e.* to nurture their children emotionally, physically and intellectually (Ruddick 1989).

> I mean I think there's a—as a mother of youngish children, you perhaps have enormous guilt and sort of think, what could you have done to prevent it? I mean you couldn't have done anything, and what are these children going to do without you? I mean it's terrible when anybody gets it but I do think it's terrible when a mother of young children has it (GC24).

Women who had grown up without a mother, or whose mother had been ill during their childhood, regarded it as particularly important to remain well until their children were adult. They talked of the importance of the mother–daughter relationship and how the presence of a mother was essential during particular rites of passage—menarche, marriage, having children etc. One woman felt the death of her mother and the loss of her support whilst she was growing up so acutely that she had already prepared a booklet for her children to read in the eventuality of her death.

> If I get it, I'm going to be organised so that my girls aren't going to forget me, or I'm not going to miss anything out, silly little things like when they're first teenagers wanting deodorants and things, I missed that as a child because my mother was too ill, she died, and there's a big growing-up gap, no matter how much different female members of the family there are, there's still that gap with a mother–daughter relationship that you've got to prepare for. I mean I know I could get run over. But I've written a little booklet (GC07).

However, these women did not just regard themselves as having a responsibility to remain healthy so that they could care for their family; they also regarded themselves as having a duty to prevent their children, or other kin, from seeing a loved one die or having to care for them. Many women, both those who had and did not have children, were still haunted by the feelings of helplessness they experienced as they watched the suffering of their mother or sister in the terminal stages of cancer, and perceived themselves as having a responsibility to do whatever was necessary to protect their relatives from such an emotional ordeal.

> Because she [mother] had a horrible death. I think she eventually suffocated and had heart failure. But when you're fifteen you're at a very impressionable age . . . no, I don't want my girls to go through that, I really don't (GC07).

Another acknowledged that it was her obligation to protect her children that influenced her decision to undergo prophylactic oophorectomy (plus hysterectomy) in spite of her fears of surgical procedures and early menopause.

> And because of my mum and dad both dying of it [cancer] within a year, and it was so horrendous . . . It really is horrible, and I wouldn't wish it on my children, to have to go through what I went through with my parents. I hate that thought, you know . . . at the end of the day you just want to be okay for your family really (GC25).

Miller (1976) observes that women's sense of self-worth is primarily based upon caring for, and giving to, others. She argues that women frequently translate their own motivations into a means of serving and caring for others. The women in this study similarly justified their willingness to adopt potentially harmful risk management practices as motivated by their obligations to fulfil others' needs: to engage in mothering work, to prevent family members from seeing them suffer or having to care for them and to provide dying relatives with peace of mind. Thus, it can be argued that these women's risk management choices are constrained by those gendered discourses which position women as responsible for the care of others, for they regard their ability to fulfil their obligations of care as dependent upon them taking steps to control their risk.

However, this does not mean that the decision to determine and manage one's cancer risks is necessarily experienced as disempowering. It must be borne in mind that many of these women felt powerless, in the face of their family history of cancer, they believed they would develop this disease in the future. But they repeatedly displaced their own needs to be cared for into an obligation to care for others. The risk of cancer was not just seen as a threat to their health, but was constructed as potentially jeopardising their ability to care for their kin and as a result, threatened their identity as carer or nurturer. Many acknowledged that a woman with cancer is unable to fulfil her obligations of care, instead of being the carer or nurturer of others she becomes the cared for and nurtured. Thus, the decision to engage in risk management was perceived as a way of counteracting the threat of cancer, and as such, as providing them with some form of control over their destiny. For these women, caring for others meant they must take steps to determine and manage their risk. By acting in this way they not only gain some control over their lives, but, more importantly, they can maintain their identity as selves-in-relation—as carers, mothers, sisters, daughters etc. (Howson 1998, Miller 1976).

## Risk management following genetic counselling

Theoretically, these women can either live with their cancer risk or take steps to define and control it. However, in reality, for most, obtaining risk information and managing cancer risk was not seen as a matter of choice, but as a matter of necessity. Therefore, given that the majority of these women were committed to taking some form of action to manage their risk so that they might fulfil their obligations to their kin, the option of no further medical intervention was effectively ruled out, even before they came to the clinic. Indeed, it can be speculated that those participants who were presented with this option during their consultation may not even have regarded it as a 'real choice' (Charles *et al.* 1998).

Thus, although the clinicians usually distinguished between best and worst case scenarios when calculating risks, and went on to make risk management recommendations on the basis of the former, with one exception, the women overlooked this distinction. During the post-clinic interview only one woman, who was told her cancer risk was low, said she intended to do nothing further about her risk. Six women said that they intended to follow the geneticists' recommendations and explore the option of prophylactic surgery (two, mastectomy and four, oophorectomy), and the remaining women said that they intended to manage their risks by joining a screening programme.

The women were interviewed a year later to establish whether they had undergone screening or surgery. With two exceptions, all those contacted had either had screening or taken steps to obtain it. As the genetics clinic they attended did not offer screening, all these women had to seek a referral for screening elsewhere. Most said they had experienced little, or no difficulty, in obtaining access to these services. As far as the two women who had decided not to pursue the option of screening were concerned, one had tried unsuccessfully to obtain ovarian screening on the NHS. She said that she had given up trying and felt less anxious about her risk now. The other—a doctor—had been advised to have annual mammography, but had decided not to pursue this because of the risks of x-rays.

One woman had seen a breast surgeon to discuss mastectomy and had postponed making a decision. All those who had said they intended to discuss oophorectomy with a gynaecologist had undergone surgery (oophorectomy plus hysterectomy) during the year following counselling. Although some were experiencing unpleasant side-effects from their hormone replacement therapy (HRT), all were satisfied that they had made the right decision, as one woman said:

> I've got no regrets about having a hysterectomy. . . .—it's the best thing I've ever had done . . . it's just—I just feel normal again. I don't, I don't think about that I'm going to die soon and I don't have all those fears any more (GC25).

Finally, one woman reported that when she attended an ovarian screening appointment she was told by her gynaecologist that she should book in for surgery in a few weeks time. She said that once she has recovered from the shock, she had decided to proceed with surgery, but had postponed the operation until the following year.

Despite the fact that all the women made it clear that they alone were responsible for the decision to manage their risks, as was noted above, there was evidence that particular forms of risk management were actively encouraged by the geneticists (Hallowell 1998a). Thus, it could be argued that the women's feelings of responsibility to their kin were not the only constraints on their risk management choices. Indeed, the labelling of these women as (potentially) 'at-risk', and the biassed presentation of risk management options during the consultations could be seen as potentially disempowering.

However, this interpretation overlooks the fact that these genetic consultations occurred within a particular social context. The way in which the clinicians discussed risk management may not have been neutral, but these women did not have a neutral agenda either. They said that they had attended the genetic clinic with the intention of doing whatever they regarded was necessary to minimise their risk so that they could fulfil their obligations to their families. It could be argued that by constructing themselves as at-risk and in need of risk management most had not only invested in, but were constrained by, the discourse of the new genetics before they attended the clinic. But this does not mean they could not, and did not, act autonomously within these constraints. Indeed, many women vigorously resisted the clinician's advice and went on to engage in risk management even when the geneticists indicated that, without confirmation of their family history, this would be inappropriate.

However, it must be noted that although the decision to manage risk may be experienced as empowering, the women in this study potentially pay a high price for assuming responsibility for their risk. All were healthy, and none had their carrier status confirmed by genetic testing, indeed, in some cases their sketchy and/or unconfirmed family history constituted what geneticists would term a non-significant pedigree. Nevertheless, following their attendance at genetic counselling, nearly all voluntarily underwent, or had arranged to undergo, medical procedures which many regarded as uncomfortable, painful or embarrassing. These procedures might not only have iatrogenic consequences, but might compromise their fertility, sexuality, body image and gender identity. In other words, by positioning themselves as 'at-risk', and taking responsibility for their genetic risk, these healthy women voluntarily put themselves at risk.

**Discussion**

Health in the late 20th century has become a matter of individual responsibility. It is assumed that a responsible individual should not only consult experts who can quantify the risks to their health and provide information about risk management, but should also act upon this advice and take steps to manage their health risks (Petersen and Lupton 1996). It has been observed that the construction of health as a moral issue is no longer only confined to discussions of voluntary health risks, but is also apparent in discussions of genetic risk (Petersen 1998). The rhetoric of the new genetics constructs individuals as having a responsibility to obtain genetic knowledge and subsequently attempt to modify their risks. This chapter has suggested that this view is not only perpetuated within the clinic (Petersen 1998), but also by at-risk individuals attending genetic counselling.

The women in the present study described themselves as having a responsibility to their kin to establish the magnitude of their risk, and the risks to other family members, and to act upon this information by engaging in some form of risk management. Thus, it was argued that the construction of risk and risk management as a moral issue constrains women's choices.

However, it could be argued that in constructing genetic risk as a moral issue these women not only limit their own choices, but potentially constrain those of others, both their lateral kin—siblings and cousins—and their descendants. These accounts demonstrate that the responsibility for determining and managing risk was transmitted not only within their own generation, but also from one generation to the next, it extended both backwards and forwards in time across the generations. These women not only saw themselves as responsible for putting their descendants at risk, but also acknowledged that they had an obligation to determine and manage their risk so that they could absolve previous generations of the responsibility for putting them at risk. Whether their relatives perceived themselves as similarly constrained by these women's actions, particularly their decision to engage in risk management, is an interesting question.

The tendency for women to position themselves as selves-in-relation (Gilligan, 1982), to see their lives as inter-connected with the lives of others, or to define themselves in terms of their social relationships with, and obligations to, others (Miller 1976, Held 1993) is well documented. Furthermore, it has long been accepted that women in general, and mothers in particular, regard themselves as bearing the responsibility for others' health and well being (Graham 1979, Ruddick 1990). In justifying their behaviour the women in this study, those who were mothers and those who were not, drew upon those gendered discourses of motherhood and womanhood which position women as responsible for care of others, not necessarily those they are biologically connected to. Thus, the extent to which the feelings of duty and obligations expressed by these women were influenced by the fact they were talking about genetic risks rather than any other type of health risk is hard to determine. Although an awareness of their biological connections may have resulted in these women feeling that they had a responsibility to determine their genetic risk, their accounts suggest that it was their acknowledgement of their social connections and associated obligations which led them to manage their own risks and to inform others about their risks and encourage them to engage in risk management. Indeed, it would be very interesting to see whether men who are faced with similar decisions account for their behaviour in a similar way.

In conclusion, the geneticisation of disease has profound implications for society in terms of how we think about the self and our bodies. It has lead to the recategorisation of the healthy as at-risk—'the potentially sick, potentially vulnerable and potentially stigmatized' (Kenen 1994: 49). Most of the women in this study had invested in this biomedical discourse before they attended the clinic—they had already positioned themselves as 'at-risk'. They had also invested in those gendered discourses which position women as responsible for the care of others and thus, were prepared to undergo (potentially risky) medical interventions to modify their at-risk status so they could fulfil their obligations of care. This construction of the self may indeed, be disempowering (Bartky 1990), and constrain women's choices (Steinberg 1996). Furthermore, the management of one's cancer risk may have considerable physical and emotional costs for the individual. However, as was apparent in their accounts, these women do not construct themselves as individuals per se, but as selves-in-relation, as interconnected to past, present and future generations. Therefore, as far as most women were concerned, obtaining genetic information about oneself and subsequently managing one's risk was seen as an intermediate goal. It was perceived as the only way in which they could ensure that they were able to fulfil their obligations to their kin—to provide them with peace of mind, practical and emotional care or genetic information. Thus, the potential costs of defining one's risks and screening/surgery were offset against the perceived benefits to others and ultimately, the indirect benefit to the self, namely the opportunity to reconfirm the self as a self-in-relation.

## Acknowledgements

I would like to thank all of the women who took part in this study, Bruce Ponder, Charis Eng, Helen Staham and Frances Murton. Many friends and colleagues have provided invaluable advice, support and encouragement during the writing of this chapter: Shelley Day Sclater, Ginny Morrow, Claire Snowdon, Gill Dunne, Frances Price and June Peters. This research was funded by the Medical Research Council Grant No. 303315 awarded to J.M. Green and M.P.M. Richards. The familial cancer clinic was supported by grants from the Cancer Research Campaign [CRC] to BAJ Ponder.

## Notes

1   This is not to deny that environmental or behavioural factors may interact with genetic factors to produce ill-health.
2   Jofesson (1998) reports that the cumulative risk of a false positive result after ten mammograms and clinical breast examinations is 49 per cent in low risk populations in the United States.
3   These risks may be ameliorated by hormone replacement therapy (HRT). However, Schrag et al. (1997) calculate that gains in life expectancy following prophylactic

oophorectomy are only valid if HRT compliance is 100 per cent. Moreover, there is an absence of data which explore the long-term effects of taking HRT.
4   An analysis of these sessions is presented in Hallowell (1998a).
5   As Chapple (1995) notes, many parents who attend genetic counselling express feelings of guilt, and blame themselves for putting their children at genetic risk.
6   Studies of men and women undergoing predictive testing for HBOC (Lerman *et al.* 1996, Watson *et al.* 1995) report that providing information for other relatives, particularly children and siblings, is perceived as one of the most important benefits of predictive testing. Similarly, Wexler (1992) reports that some individuals undergo DNA-testing for Huntington's disease purely for altruistic reasons *i.e.* to provide information for other family members.
7   Similar observations have been made by Kerr *et al.* (1998), who report that their participants cited altruism as a major motivation for taking part in clinical research.

# References

Backett, K. (1992) Taboos and excesses: lay moralities in middle class families. *Sociology of Health and Illness*, 14, 255–74.

Baric, I. (1969) Recognition of the 'at-risk' role: a means to influence health behaviour, *International Journal of Health Education*, 12, 24–34.

Bartky, S.L. (1990) *Femininity and Domination: Studies in the Phenomenology of Oppression*. New York: Routledge.

Burke, W., Daly, M., Garber, J., Botkin, J., Kahn, M.J. and Lynch, P. (1997) Recommendations for follow-up care of individuals with an inherited predisposition to cancer II. BRCA1 and BRCA2, *Journal of the American Medical Association*, 277, 997–1003.

Castel, R. (1991) From dangerousness to risk. In Burchell, G. and Miller, P. (eds) *The Foucault Effect: Studies in Governmentality*. Hemel Hempstead: Harvester Wheatsheaf.

Chapple, A. (1995) Parental guilt: the part played by the clinical geneticist, *Journal of Genetic Counseling*, 4, 179–91.

Charles, C., Redko, C., Whelan, T., Gafni, A. and Reyno, L. (1998) Doing nothing is no choice: lay constructions of treatment decision-making among women with early stage breast cancer, *Sociology of Health and Illness*, 20, 1, 71–95.

Cooper, C. and Dennison, E. (1998) Do silicon breast implants cause connective tissue disease? *British Medical Journal*, 316, 403–4.

Crawford, R. (1977) You are dangerous to your health: the ideology and politics of victim blaming, *International Journal of Health Services*, 7, 663–80.

Den Otter, W., Merchant, T.E., Beijerinck, D. and Kotten, J.W. (1996) Breast cancer induction due to mammographic screening in hereditary *Anticancer Research*, 16, 3173–6.

Douglas, M. (1992) *Risk and Blame: Essays in Cultural Theory*. London: Routledge.

Douglas, M. and Wildavsky, A. (1982) *Risk and Culture*. Berkley: University of California Press.

Easton, D.F., Ford, D., Bishop, D.T. and the Breast Cancer Linkage Consortium. (1995) Breast and ovarian cancer incidence in BRCA1 mutation carriers, *American Journal of Human Genetics*, 56, 265–71.

Gilligan, C. (1982) *In a Different Voice: Psychological Theory and Women's Development*. London: Harvard University Press.

Graham, H. (1979) 'Prevention and health: every mother's business': a comment on child health policies in the 1970s. In Harris, C. (ed) *The Sociology of the Family: New Directions for Britain*. Keele: Sociological Review Monograph, 28.

Hallowell, N. (1998a) Genetic risks and responsibilities: or how the neutrality of genetic counselling is compromised. Paper presented at the 14th World Congress of Sociology, Montreal, 26 July–1 August.

Hallowell, N. (1998b) Risk management following genetic testing: women's information needs. Paper presented at the Fifth International Meeting on the Psychosocial Aspects of Genetic Testing for Hereditary Breast and/or Ovarian Cancer. Leuven, 29th–30th June.

Hallowell, N. (1999) Reconstructing the body or reconstructing the woman? Perceptions of prophylactic mastectomy for hereditary breast cancer risk. In Potts, L. (ed) *Ideologies of Breast Cancer*. London: Macmillan Press. *(Forthcoming)*.

Hartmann, L., Jenkins, R., Schaid, D. and Yang, P. (1997) Prophylactic mastectomy: preliminary retrospective cohort analysis, *Proceedings of the American Association for Cancer Research*, 38, 168.

Held, V. (1993) *Feminist Morality*. Chicago and London: University of Chicago Press.

Howson, A. (1998) Embodied obligation: the female body and health surveillance. In Nettleton, S. and Watson, J. (eds) *The Body in Everyday Life*. London and New York: Routledge.

Jofesson, D. (1998) High risk of false positives with breast screening, *British Medical Journal*, 316, 1261–2.

Kash, K., Holland, J.C., Halper, M.S. and Miller, D.G. (1992) Psychological distress and surveillance behaviours of women with a family history of breast cancer, *Journal of the National Cancer Institute*, 84, 24–30.

Katz Rothman, B. (1994) *The Tentative Pregnancy: Amniocentesis and the Sexual Politics of Motherhood*. London: Pandora.

Kenen, R. (1994) The Human Genome Project: creator of the potentially sick, potentially vulnerable and potentially stigmatized? In Robinson, I. (ed) *Life and Death under High Technology Medicine*. Manchester: Manchester University Press.

Kerr, A., Cunningham-Burley, S. and Amos, A. (1998) The new genetics and health: mobilizing lay expertise, *Public Understanding of Science*. 7, 41–60.

Kerr, A. and Cunningham-Burley, S. (1998) On ambivalence and risk: professional and lay accounts of the new genetics. Mimeo. Department of Public Health Sciences, University of Edinburgh.

Lerman, C. and Schwartz, M. (1993) Adherence and psychological adjustment among women at high risk for breast cancer, *Breast Cancer Research and Treatment*, 28, 145–55.

Lerman, C., Narod, S., Sculman, K., Hughes, C., Gomez-Carminero, A. and Bonney, G. (1996) BRCA1 testing in families with Hereditary Breast–Ovarian cancer, *Journal of the American Medical Association*, 275, 1885–92.

Lippman, A. (1992) Led (astray) by genetic maps: the cartography of the human genome and healthcare, *Social Science and Medicine*, 35, 1469–76.

Lippmann-Hand, A. and Fraser, C. (1979a) Genetic counselling: provision and reception of information, *American Journal of Medical Genetics*, 3, 113–27.

Lippmann-Hand, A. and Fraser, C. (1979b) Genetic counselling: parents' responses to uncertainty, *Birth Defects Original Articles Series*, 15, 325–39.

Lupton, D. (1993) Risk as moral danger: the social and political functions of risk discourse in public health, *International Journal of Health Services*, 23, 425–35.

Lupton, D. (1995) *The Imperative of Health: Public Health and the Regulated Body*. London: Sage.

Mason, J. (1996) Gender, care and sensibility in family and kin relationships. In Holland, J. and Adkins, L. (eds) *Sex, Sensibility and the Gendered Body*. Basingstoke: Macmillan.

Miki, J., Swensen, J., Shattuck-Eidens, D., Futreal, P.A., Hershman, K., Tavigian, S., *et al.* (1994) A strong candidate for the breast ovarian cancer susceptibility gene BRCA1, *Science*, 266, 66–71.

Miller, J.B. (1976) *Toward a New Psychology of Women*. London: Allen Lane.

Muhr, T. (1994) *Atlas-ti: Computer aided Text Interpretation and Theory Building*. Berlin: Self Published.

National Institute of Health Consensus Conference Statement (1994) Ovarian cancer: screening, treatment, and follow-up, *Gynecological Oncology*, 55, S4–14.

Neugut, A.I. and Jacobson, J.S. (1995) The limitations of breast cancer screening for first degree relatives of breast cancer patients, *American Journal of Public Health*, 85, 832–4.

Odets, W. (1995) *In the Shadow of the Epidemic: Being HIV-negative in the Age of AIDS*. London: Cassell.

Parsons, E. and Atkinson, P. (1992) Lay constructions of genetic risk, *Sociology of Health and Illness,* 14, 437–55.

Parsons, E. and Clarke, A.J. (1993) Genetic risk: women's understanding of carrier risks in Duchenne muscular dystrophy, *Journal of Medical Genetics,* 30, 562–6.

Patton, C. (1993) 'With champagne and roses': women at risk from/in AIDS discourse. In Squires, C. (ed) *Women and AIDS: Psychological Perspectives*. London: Sage.

Pearn, J.H. (1973) Patients' subjective interpretation of risks offered in genetic counselling, *Journal of Medical Genetics,* 10, 129–34.

Pernet, A.J., Wardle, J., Bourne, T.H., Whitehead, M.I., Campbell, S. and Collins, W.P. (1992) A qualitative evaluation of the experience of surgery after false ositive results in screening for familial ovarian cancer, *Psycho-Oncology*, 1, 217–33.

Petersen, A. (1998) The new genetics and the politics of public health, *Critical Public Health*, 8, 59–72.

Petersen, A. and Lupton, D. (1996) *The New Public Health: Health and Self in the Age of Risk*. London: Sage.

Pill, R. and Stott, N.C.H. (1982) Concepts of illness causation and responsibility: some preliminary data from a sample of working class mothers, *Social Science and Medicine*, 16, 43–52.

Piver, M.S., Jishi, M.F., Tsukada, Y. and Nava, G. (1993) Primary peritoneal carcinoma after prophylactic oophorectomy in women with a family history of ovarian cancer. A report of the Gilda Radner Familial Ovarian Cancer Registry, *Cancer*, 71, 2751–5.

Ruddick, S. (1989) *Maternal Thinking: Towards a Politics of Peace*. London: The Women's Press.

Schrag, D., Kuntz, K.M., Garber, J. and Weeks, J.C. (1997) Decision analysis—effects of prophylactic mastectomy and oophorectomy on life expectancy among women with *BRCA1* or *BRCA2* mutations, *New England Journal of Medicine*, 336, 1465–71.

Steinberg, D.L. (1996) Languages of risk: genetic encryptions of the female body, *women: a Cultural Review*, 7, 259–70.

Stephanek, M.E., Helzlsouer, K.J., Wilcox, P.M. and Houn, F. (1995) Predictors of and satisfaction with bilateral prophylactic mastectomy, *Preventative Medicine*, 24, 412–19.

Tobacman, J.K., Greene, M.H., Tucker, M.A., Costa, J., Kase, R. and Fraumeni, J.F.Jr. (1982) Intra-abdominal carcinomatosis after prophylactic oophorectomy in ovarian-cancer-prone families, *Lancet*, ii, 195–9.

Tong, R. (1997) *Feminist Approaches to Bioethics: Theoretical Reflections and Practical Applications*. Oxford: Westview Press.

Tonin, P., Ghadirian, P., Phelan, C., Lenoir, G.M., Lynch, H.T. and Letendre, F. (1995) A large multisite cancer family is linked to BRCA2, *Journal of Medical Genetics*, 32, 982–4.

Wardle, J. (1995) Women at risk of ovarian cancer, *Journal of the National Cancer Institute Monographs*, 17, 81–5.

Watson, M., Murday, V., Lloyd, S., *et al.* (1995) Genetic testing in breast/ovarian cancer (BRCA1) families, *Lancet*, 346, 583.

Wexler, N.S. (1992) Clairvoyance and caution: repercussions of the Human Genome Project. In Kevles, D.J. and Wood, L. (eds) *The Code of Codes: Scientific and Social Issues in the Human Genome Project*. Cambridge, Mass. and London: Harvard University Press.

Wooster, R., Neuhausen, S., Mangion, J., Quirk, Y., Ford, D. and Collins, N. (1994) Localisation of a breast cancer susceptibility gene (BRCA2) to chromosome 13q by linkage analysis, *Science*, 265, 2088–90.

Ziegler, L.D. and Kroll, S.S. (1991) Primary breast cancer after prophylactic mastectomy, *American Journal of Clinical Oncology*, 14, 451–4.

# 'There's this thing in our family': predictive testing and the construction of risk for Huntington Disease

## Susan M. Cox and William McKellin

---

### Introduction

Recent discussions about the social implications of the new genetics stress the importance of studying hereditary risk within the context of familial beliefs and dynamics (Hayes 1992, Kessler and Bloch 1989, Richards, M. 1993). Empirical studies on predictive testing have, however, focused primarily on the psychological implications of receiving an informative test result. Few studies examine how test candidates and their families jointly construct the meaning of hereditary risk within their everyday lives and how, in turn, such pre-existing constructions shape the experience of predictive testing.

This chapter examines the social construction of hereditary risk for Huntington Disease. HD is an adult-onset autosomal dominant neuropsychiatric disorder. There is no effective prevention or cure, but through predictive testing, it is possible to determine whether or not at-risk individuals have inherited the genetic mutation associated with HD.

In contrast with studies which examine representations of hereditary risk in science and medicine (Nelkin and Lindee 1995, Nukaga and Cambrosio 1997, Yoxen 1982) or the communicative interactions of the genetics clinic (Press and Browner 1997, Rapp 1988), this chapter emphasises the intersubjective construction of risk within the everyday and 'everynight' (Smith 1987) worlds of test candidates and their families. Given that many service providers tend to assume that a priori risk is subjectively interpreted in a relatively uniform way, lay understandings of risk are often neglected within the predominantly rational clinical discourse on the potential costs and benefits of genetic testing (Boutté 1988, Press and Browner 1997).

Drawing upon Bloor's (1995) analytic approach to HIV-related risk behaviours, we suggest that an adequate theoretical scheme for understanding how lay actors interpret hereditary risk and its modification through predictive testing must encompass the 'world of routine activities' (Schutz 1967) as well as the world of considered alternatives. It must eschew the assumption that hereditary risk has a constant and/or high degree of relevance and, instead, prompt inquiry into how the 'state of being at risk' (Lippman-Hand and Fraser 1979) is, over time, constituted by test candidates (and their significant others) as both problematic *and* amenable to strategic intervention (*i.e.* predictive testing). Finally, this scheme must also embrace the socially constrained as well as volitional character of cognition (Bloor 1995) showing how, in the absence of an appropriate popular discourse on hereditary and other forms of embodied risk (Kavanagh and Broom 1998), lay actors adapt and modify culturally available frameworks in order to interpret hereditary risk in an intersubjectively meaningful way (Bourdieu 1977).

The research locale is extremely important in this: the stories that people tell when they are 'probands',[1] patients or clients in the clinic, differ from the stories that people tell when they are at home, work or otherwise living their lives (Burgess submitted). In particular, the range of elements which have topical and interpretive relevance are different. As Conrad argues more generally:

> Much research on illness experience has assumed that studying patient-hood from the patient's perspective—especially doctor–patient inter-action—is the same as studying illness experience. It is not (1990: 1260).

Researchers must go beyond clinical settings in order to focus on how at risk individuals and their families understand hereditary risk in everyday life. This shift points to significant lacunae for sociological investigation—from the salient differences between lay and scientific constructions of hereditary risk (Parsons and Atkinson 1992, Richards and Ponder 1996) to the gendered division of labour that characterises familial patterns of communication about the family history of hereditary disease (Cox 1998, 1999, Green *et al.* 1997, Shakespeare 1992). Moreover, it raises the possibility of doing research that gives priority to the needs of at risk individuals and their families, rather than service providers.

Here, we focus on the social, biographical and temporal factors central to lay understandings of hereditary risk and its modification through predictive testing. Mendelian theories of inheritance[2] stress the random nature of gene transmission and offer an objective calculus for describing a priori risk. This abstract form of knowledge is, however, inadequate for conceptualising the lived experience of risk as it develops within the nexus of familial relations. As Gifford proposes, lay risk is 'not objective, cannot be quantified or measured, and is not static', it 'must be understood as a dynamic experience of personal uncertainty' about one's own and, we would add, one's family members' future (1986: 230).

## Huntington Disease and predictive testing

Huntington Disease (HD) poses stark questions about the social meanings of hereditary risk. It is a degenerative neuropsychiatric disorder characterised by involuntary movements, personality changes, cognitive impairment, and depression. Onset typically occurs in mid-life (between the ages of

35 and 45), although much earlier and later occurrences are known (Hayden 1981). The gradual but inexorable progression of the disease varies, but death usually occurs 15 to 20 years after onset. Because of its typical late onset, it is described as a 'genetic time bomb' which 'remains dormant until the person reaches adulthood' (Huntington Society of Canada 1996).

As an *autosomal dominant*, HD affects, and is transmitted to the next generation, by both sexes. All offspring of an affected individual therefore have a 50 per cent chance of inheriting the mutation associated with HD; this is a random event which is often compared to the 'flip of a coin'. The mutation is highly *penetrant*; thus anyone who inherits it will, if they live long enough, almost certainly become affected. Not inheriting the mutation—an equally chance event—means that the 'chain is broken' and that HD will not reappear in subsequent generations.

The first symptoms of HD are often a source of anxiety and uncertainty for at-risk individuals and their families (Hayes 1992, Kessler 1993, Kessler and Bloch 1989, Wexler 1979). Prior to the development of predictive testing, such uncertainty could only be resolved through clinical diagnosis. With the 1983 discovery of a linked marker for the HD gene a presymptomatic test was developed. As the first proof of the power of new techniques in gene mapping, this discovery was highly significant to the human genetics and molecular biology communities (Wexler 1995).

In 1986, centres in Canada, the U.S. and U.K. began to offer the linkage test. Given concerns about the potentially catastrophic effects of hearing an increased risk result, the test protocol included extensive psychosocial assessment and counselling (Brandt *et al.* 1989, Fox *et al.* 1989). With the 1993 discovery of the mutation associated with HD, a definitive or 'direct' predictive test was developed (Goldberg *et al.* 1993, Huntington's Disease Collaborative Research Group 1993). In contrast with linkage testing, the direct test is based upon analysis of the region of DNA believed to be directly implicated in causing HD. This region—which is located on the short arm of chromosome 4—has been described as a 'genetic stutter' (Hayden 1993) in which the trinucleotide sequence of CAG is repeated many more times than in the unaffected population.[3]

With direct testing, at-risk individuals learn that they have inherited a normal allele (35 or fewer CAG repeats) *or* an expanded allele (42 or more CAG repeats). Further, a very small number two to three per cent) learn they have an intermediate allele (36 to 41 CAG repeats): such individuals may or *may not* develop HD within a normal life span thus the gene may, in some cases, have reduced penetrance (Brinkman *et al.* 1997).

**Study design**

The findings presented here derive from a prospective qualitative study of the social meanings and lived experiences of predictive testing for HD. In

British Columbia, the site of this study, predictive testing is guided by the following criteria: the test candidate must (1) have a confirmed family history of HD and an a priori risk of 50 or 25 per cent; (2) be able to provide informed consent; and (3) not have been diagnosed with HD. Predictive testing is, therefore, 'only for persons who consider themselves to be at risk' for, but not yet affected by, the onset of HD (Benjamin *et al.* 1994: 607). Thus far, only 10 to 15 per cent of persons at risk for HD have requested predictive testing.

In our study, the genetic counsellor assisted in recruitment by providing all new test candidates with information about our research. We met interested test candidates at the clinic, and those who agreed to take part in the study selected other family members to participate with them. Over a 10-month period (1993–1994) we obtained a sample of 22 predictive test candidates (from 21 different families) and 41 family members from urban and rural settings (see Table 1). This sample represents 81 per cent of all new test candidates seen at the clinic during this period. Three test candidates had obtained an informative test result through prior participation in linkage testing (two had a decreased risk and one an increased risk). None withdrew from predictive testing for this research prior to learning their direct test results.

Our sample reflects two widely reported patterns in predictive testing: (1) the ratio of female to male test candidates is approximately 2 : 1,[4] and (2) the number of test candidates who do not have the mutation is nearly double the number who have the mutation[5] (see Table 2). Background information on all study participants cited in this chapter is contained in Table 3.[6]

Table 1: *Distribution of Family Members*

| Relationship of Family Members to Predictive Test Candidate | | | |
|---|---|---|---|
| Spouse/Partners | 16 | Wife/Female | 6 |
| | | Husband/Male | 10 |
| Parents | 3 | Mother | 2 |
| | | Father | 1 |
| Siblings | 9 | Sister | 4 |
| | | Brother | 5 |
| Children | 4 | Daughter | 2 |
| | | Son | 2 |
| Other Family | 6 | Female | 5 |
| | | Male | 1 |
| Friends | 3 | Female | 3 |
| | | Male | 0 |
| Total Family Members | 41 | Female | 22 |
| | | Male | 19 |

Table 2:  *Test Results of Predictive Test Candidates by Gender*

| | *Total Number of Predictive Test Candidates = 22* | | |
| | *Do Not Have Gene for HD* | *Intermediate Allele* | *Have Gene for HD* |
|---|---|---|---|
| Female | 8 | 1 | 6 |
| Male | 6 | 0 | 1 |
| | 14 | 1 | 7 |

Data collection took place from 1993 to 1997. In-depth interviews were conducted individually in participants' homes several weeks before and four to eight months after disclosure of the test results. Six families also participated in a third round of interviews conducted approximately two years after results. These interviews covered a consistent set of topics but participants were encouraged to talk about what *they* felt was most important and to frame this in whatever ways seemed most appropriate to them. This approach enhanced validity by allowing participants to pattern the timing, sequence, content, and context of topics discussed (Mishler 1991). Interviews lasted from one to three hours and were tape recorded and transcribed. The qualitative software programme NUD.IST (Richards 1994, Richards and Richards 1994) was employed in the management and thematic analysis of the data. Analysis proceeded in an iterative fashion as we developed and refined our understanding of the patterns which emerged from participants' narrative accounts. This process yielded new insight into familial constructions of hereditary risk, patterns of communication, experiences of predictive testing and interpretations of clinical information.

**The relevance of risk**

Though it is now recognised that most families at risk for dominantly inherited disorders are aware of the family history as well as the etiology and genetics of the disease (Richards 1993), there are few studies which consider how such awareness emerges. Moreover, much of the literature on HD suggests that hereditary risk is a source of protracted anxiety. Drawing upon Schutz's (1970) system of relevances, we suggest that it ought not to be taken for granted by social scientists (or clinicians) that hereditary risk is inherently problematic; to do so is to assume that which is in need of explanation.

Schutz (1946) distinguishes several 'zones of relevance' which reflect the fluctuating 'interests at hand' of lay actors. These zones form a continuum that is distinguished by the degree of certitude, knowledge and considered action required of lay actors confronted with a theoretical or practical problem. This system of interests and their priorisation in various zones of

Table 3: *Background Information on Study Participants Cited in Text*

| Pseudonym | Gender | Status[1] | A priori risk[2] | Age | Marital status | Children[3] |
|---|---|---|---|---|---|---|
| Jason | Male | son | 25 | 29 | single | 0 |
| Gabriella | Female | PTC | 50 | 54 | married | 2 |
| Maggie | Female | PTC | 50 | 57 | married | 5 |
| Rosalind | Female | PTC | 50 | 57 | married | 2 |
| Helen | Female | PTC | 25 | 47 | common-law | 3 |
| Duane | Male | husband | n/a | 43 | married | 3 |
| Landis | Female | PTC & sister | 50 | 28 | single | 0 |
| Nigel | Male | PTC & brother | 50 | 29 | single | 0 |
| Heather | Female | PTC | 50 | 34 | married | 2 |
| Mitchell | Male | father | Dx | 47 | married | 2 |
| Colin | Male | PTC | 50 | 41 | married | 3 |
| Emily | Female | wife | n/a | 39 | married | 3 |
| Regina | Female | PTC | 50 | 28 | married | 1 |
| Albert | Male | PTC | 50 | 46 | single | 0 |
| Anne | Female | PTC | 50 | 46 | married | 2 |
| Michael | Male | PTC | 50 | 45 | married | 2 |
| Peter | Male | husband | n/a | 46 | married | 0 |

[1] *Status* indicated by the abbreviation PTC to designate a predictive test candidate or another descriptor (*e.g.* son) indicating the relationship of the study participant to the PTC.

[2] *A priori risk* is expressed as a percentage; the abbreviation Dx designates a study participant who is diagnosed with HD; the abbreviation n/a designates a study participant who is not and has never been at risk for HD.

[3] The *number of children* includes all children (*i.e.* biologically and non-biologically related).

relevance is neither constant nor homogeneous; there is always a plurality of interests with some topical relevance and an array of elements which have interpretive and motivational relevance (Schutz 1970).

The fluidity of these interests is particularly important when considering the fluctuating relevance of hereditary risk throughout the life course. In their study of women's assessments of carrier status and risk for Duchenne Muscular Dystrophy,[7] Parsons and Atkinson (1992) demonstrate that information about risk is retained in a zone of high relevance at certain critical junctures (*e.g.* decisions about marriage or reproduction). Where carrier risk status is not experienced as discrediting, it may, at other times, assume a characteristic latency.

Though the potential for such periods of 'latency' differs substantially for persons at risk of HD, our findings suggest that the relevance of risk is nonetheless fluid and contingent: information about risk is, at certain critical junctures, given a high degree of relevance while at other times, it has much less importance. The diagnosis of HD in a parent or sibling often constitutes one such critical juncture while the decision to request predictive testing constitutes another: both raise the potential for the objective modification of a priori risk but, more centrally, both are moments in which everyday routines are disrupted and hereditary risk becomes a topic of discussion.

Here we wish to acknowledge that some study participants said that their involvement in our research led them to think and talk more extensively about hereditary risk. This was especially germane to family members who had *not* attended pre-test genetic counselling sessions. Further, it illustrates how research on such sensitive issues is inevitably an intervention in, as well as an attempt to understand, the intersubjective realities of test candidates and their families (Lee 1993). Talking is, after all, a means of allocating things a definite place in the world and conversation is, therefore, an important vehicle of reality-construction and maintenance. As Berger and Luckman propose, 'language realizes a world, in the double sense of apprehending and producing it' (1966: 174).

*'This thing in our family'*
How does hereditary risk become the subject of considered attention? As suggested by the title of this chapter, HD is often referred to by at-risk individuals as 'this thing' that is 'in' the family; it is unnamed, not because it is, like cancer, somehow unmentionable (Frank 1991), but because it is, at times, a diffuse part of the taken-for-granted knowledge which informs family life. 'This thing' is, however, also complex and, in keeping with the way that complex objects are often represented (in English) by their containers (Reddy 1993), 'this thing' is an object that is represented by way of its' containment within the family.

Jason was typical of those who recalled having an early but diffuse awareness of HD. His mother was at 50 per cent a priori risk. When asked about his first recollections of learning there was a family history of HD, Jason said:

Somewhere about grade seven we used to have [Huntington Society] meetings at our house . . . There were a few people with Huntington's there . . . I was around, I didn't shy away from it but I wasn't really a participant . . . I don't think we ever avoided the issue but I don't remember a day in my life when (my parents) sat me down and said, 'look son, there's thing thing in our family' so I don't know when it started.

It was not until Jason's mother requested predictive testing that Jason began to seriously consider his own genetic status. Near the end of the pre-results interview, he said:

It brings up strange emotions now that we talk so specifically about it [my risk] . . . and about predictive testing cos I've always thought 'well I'll do that some day or I might have to do that some day' but I've never actually pinpointed . . . when I would do that. And now that I think about it and now that my mother is going through the test, I realise 'hey it might be now, it might be in the next two years. It might be darn close.' And that brings some odd feelings.

Maggie also grew up with some awareness of HD but did not initially know what 'it' was:

My sister and I were talking about that [our awareness of HD] and we figured we might have been 16 (pause) 17 . . . when we thought of it and saw that it was in the family. When I was I'd say closer to really knowing that it was there I was 27 . . . My Dad came to visit me . . . and he would sit there and (sound of fingers scratching on the table) you could see the scratch, scratch, and his feet were shuffling under the table (muffled sound of feet moving) all the time and it just sent me up the wall . . . We, I knew something was wrong and I guess it had been mentioned somewhere in the family that Huntington's was there but it didn't penetrate to us at the time cause we didn't know what it really was. You know, 'this old person got Huntington's.' We didn't realise it was a hereditary disease or anything. So I was somewhere between 17 and 27 before it really sunk in, I think, for me.

For Maggie, the knowledge that HD was 'in the family' didn't really 'penetrate'. Given that Maggie's father died from unrelated causes before being diagnosed with HD, the issue of hereditary risk did not surface until Maggie's younger brother experienced onset.

I didn't really worry. As I said basically it's been something in my background. It's just way there (waving hand over shoulder) and its not bothering me too much. Now it's getting a little closer because [my brother] has it . . . and with all the kids and grandkids I'm a bit worried about it.

In contrast, Rosalind received 'a real surprise' when she learned, at age 50, that her younger sister had been diagnosed with HD. Given that Rosalind's mother died from unrelated causes and her father was in his late 70s and showing no signs of HD, the hereditary nature and origin of the disease was unclear. As Rosalind recalled:

> I know of Huntington's Chorea . . . but I didn't know very much about it other than chorea, to me, was spastic, uncontrollable action. . . . And I felt that it would be something rather debilitating if it was neurological . . . but I didn't know at the time when [my sister] was diagnosed that it was genetic.

When a geneticist explained the characteristic pattern of inheritance associated with HD, Rosalind immediately took note.

> As soon as I knew that it was a genetic problem I figured well then we'd all better sit up straight and pay attention because we all could be in for some unpleasant news.

Helen also became aware of HD in mid-life when her overseas cousin mentioned, in a letter, that his sister had been diagnosed with HD. As Helen recalled:

> There was never any information coming from [Britain]. . . . I think my mother suspected that what my cousin had was hereditary, from her mother, but there was no way of confirming it. . . . We [my sister and I] didn't pay much attention to it. I mean we were all, 'well, what the hell? These are all strangers.'

Prior to her cousin's letter, Helen had never heard of HD. Both parents died from unrelated causes and, because she lived in a remote community, it was difficult to obtain information. Her local doctor did not know much about HD so she went to the library.

> If you've ever gone to a small town library, into the medical books, it is not pleasant. I came out of there and the one thing that really stuck in my head was the fact that they really didn't know what the normal cause of death was because most people [with HD] committed suicide . . . that was the one thing I learned from my little foray into the library . . . and I kind of bounced off the wall for a few days.

### 'It might be darn close'

As the preceding examples suggest, there are many interwoven social, biographical and temporal factors which shape and differentiate the relevance of hereditary risk. What each example has in common, however, is reference to a change that brings risk into the 'here and now' (Berger and Luckmann 1966).

Such changes are represented linguistically through a coherent system of orientational metaphors. These 'metaphors we live by' (Lakoff and Johnson 1980) provide an interpretive resource which lay actors draw upon to convey a sense of how hereditary risk becomes the subject of considered attention. Through this system of orientational metaphors, hereditary risk is located within the family and within a temporal flow of events. This flow of events stretches forward and back in time; it is spatialised and, within the time–space continuum, proximity conveys strength of effect (Lakoff and Johnson 1980).

This system of metaphors holds across many domains and it is the basis of how we experience and represent the social and biological relations of kinship. As Schneider (1980) demonstrates, cultural beliefs about kinship, procreation and heredity are expressions of social values and moral rela-tionships as well as biological connectedness. We say, for instance, that we have a 'close' family or that someone is a 'distant' relative. Alternatively, heredity is depicted in medical genetics through the use of symbols in a pedi-gree; some symbols are drawn in close proximity to each other and/or are connected with a vertical or horizontal line which signifies, respectively, bio-logical descent or sibship. The experience of kinship does not, however, coincide with these representations because kinship is not ordered simply in terms of biological inheritance. One consequence is that lay understandings of heredity conflict with theories of Mendelian genetics: as Richards and Ponder demonstrate, 'perceived closeness in inherited (genetic) terms' is shaped by 'the closeness of the family ties of social and emotional relation-ship and of obligation, duty, responsibility' (1996: 1033).

Let us briefly consider the heuristic value of such orientational metaphors in elucidating how hereditary risk becomes the subject of considered atten-tion. When risk is in the 'background' it has a low degree of relevance; it is a taken-for-granted aspect of everyday life that does not merit special consid-eration. As it 'comes closer', risk becomes problematic and those who are 'at' risk apprehend the change in terms of their proximity to and/or immi-nent arrival at a place of risk. This embodied as well as cognitive experience entails movement and fluidity. It is very different from having an objectified knowledge of a priori risk, so different that, following Lippman-Hand and Fraser (1979), we wish to distinguish the abstract phrase 'at risk' (as it is used within the lexicon of Mendelian genetics) from the intersubjective awareness and existential state of being 'at' risk.

Though Maggie did not mention that her brother's diagnosis was a de facto modification of her a priori risk,[8] she experienced an altered sense of proximity to HD. Risk started 'getting a little closer'; it became a more tan-gible presence within her family. Likewise, Jason implied that his mother's imminent test results posed the possibility of an objective change in his a priori risk, but he expressed the anticipated change in terms of an altered spatial–temporal proximity to hereditary risk—'it might be now . . . it might be darn close'. In contrast, neither Rosalind nor Helen knew anything about

HD until mid-life. Both described the impact of their sudden awareness through metaphors which mapped an embodied experience (of being on high alert or feeling extreme agitation) onto the more abstract domain of modes of cognition. Rosalind figured that she had better 'sit up straight' and 'pay attention' while Helen 'bounded off the wall'.

Though it is beyond the scope of this chapter to describe the social construction of HD, it is important to note that perceptions of HD differ widely according to factors which cannot be adequately conceptualised in terms of an individualistic biomedical model (Kessler and Bloch 1989). HD means many things and these meanings are often articulated by way of contrast with other more common diseases or threats. Wexler (1979) found that in contrast with the sense of unpredictability which denotes multiple sclerosis, HD imposes a burden of anticipation and silent apprehension. In our study, we observed three uses of such comparisons. Given that HD is still not a well-known disease, some participants said they likened HD to a hybrid of Alzheimer's and Parkinson's in order to render it subjectively meaningful to others. Many participants also contrasted the gradual progression of HD with the imagined horrors of HIV/AIDS or cancer in order to define a worse-case scenario. Others mentioned sudden heart attacks or being hit by a bus to underscore the fact that no-one is immortal. The future can suddenly be taken away from any one of us.

The most salient aspect of these constructions is that HD imposes a time frame. There are two related aspects to this, each of which acts in concert. The first has to do with families' intersubjective constructions of the typical age of onset. There is wide variation in the age of onset and where HD is observed to affect family members relatively late in life, it does not seem to impose such an immediate threat. Landis recalled that here awareness of HD began with her grandmother's eccentric behaviour:

> I don't have any recollection of anybody explaining it to me. It was just like, 'your grandmother has Huntington's. It's like Alzheimer's or Parkinson's.' . . . and then maybe a couple of years later having Dad say 'Well, okay, you can't get it unless one of your parents has it. If one of your parents has it you have a 50 per cent chance of getting it.' And I still don't recall it having any great impact on me whatsoever.

Shortly before we began this research, Landis's father learned that he had inherited the mutation associated with HD. Landis was concerned for her father but, because of the family history of relatively late onset, her own risk remained 'a bit of a non-issue'.

> I mean if I was to be told . . . there's a pretty good chance it's something that's going to affect you in your 30s or 40s, yeah, then I'll get interested in it. But I haven't been given any information along those lines at all and again . . . I feel like I have a lot of time.

Heather did not feel as if she had much time. When asked how she experienced the news of her mother's diagnosis she said:

> I got on it really quickly . . . we were thinking of a second child at the time and knowing that my mother had developed Huntington's around her mid-30s, and I was 31, I wanted to find out as quickly as possible where we stood. We had financial commitments, a mortgage. I'm a major wage-earner in the family. We wanted another child . . . so my concern was 'would I be a candidate [to develop HD] in my mid-30s?'

The second aspect of temporality salient to understanding the fluctuating relevance of risk has to do with the normal course of ageing and experience of durée. The transition from youthfulness to maturity is marked by a change in the lived experience of temporality. As Schutz suggests, we move from 'experiencing our future as an undisclosed open horizon of the present . . . toward the feeling of our finity' (1970: 181).

The significance of this was especially striking in what parents had to say about telling their children about HD. Where a parent has just been diagnosed, the news potentially carries a double-significance: it signals a change in the parent's health status and, simultaneously, increases the child's a priori risk from 25 to 50 per cent. These aspects do not, however, always have an equivalent relevance to parents and their children.

When Mitchell was diagnosed with HD, he and his wife explained the disease to their two teenage sons: their responses surprised him.

> When we told them what the scoop was . . . they said 'well you're old and I'm young and it's never going to happen to me.' Like that was their attitude. That I'm a dad and they're a kid. There's going to be a lot of years before they're my age and so don't worry about it.

Colin was also in his mid-teens when he learned that his father had been diagnosed with HD: he understood that he was at 50 per cent risk but he didn't worry about it because 'younger people tend to be invincible'. Happily married with three children, Colin and his wife Emily had always lived according to the philosophy that you should enjoy life as you go. Colin explained:

> You live by faith for one thing and why dwell on it? . . . But I was in my early 30s then so life has a different perspective. And then you get to 40 and I think as part of being 40 you start to look at life, whether you've got this hanging over your head or not, I still think you start to look at where you've been and where you want to go and make any course adjustments that you have to.

As Colin approached the age at which his father experienced onset (i.e. early 40s), he and Emily became increasingly aware of how HD had infiltrated everyday life. As Emily recalled:

I had concerns about Colin a year ago. He was just acting really weird . . .
And I was really scared cos I thought 'what is going on with him?' . . .
And so I spoke to my Dad and asked him . . . 'Have you noticed that
Colin's different?' 'No.' He didn't notice anything. He said 'it's just your
imagination cos you know that it's time. You're just looking for things.'
And I think maybe I was.

Family members often monitor the behaviour of at-risk individuals (Kessler
and Bloch 1989) and knowing that 'it is time' redoubles these efforts. Colin
knew that Emily was worried so he refrained from sharing his own doubts
about whether he was experiencing onset. Summing up his experience of
how risk became increasingly problematic, Colin said:

The Huntington's cloud was gathering on the horizon and it was getting
closer and closer and started hovering over me . . . I didn't think about it
heavily every day but [pause] more and more days you're thinking about
your risk situation and how it may affect your future and having your
own business you have to plan ahead and . . . you're thinking all these
things and my thinking went from not wanting the test at all to at least
getting my blood banked to thinking that maybe I would get the test so
that I can use it as an instrument for planning my future.

Colin does, in his words, a '180 degree turn' and moves from not wanting
to consider predictive testing to deciding that the test is an 'instrument' he
can *use* in planning the future. As such, he reframes his own sense of
agency. As he said:

It took me a long time to decide I wanted to do it. I had to evolve towards
it but I can lift the cloud.

Here Colin acknowledges that his 'risk situation' is both problematic and
amenable to strategic intervention: it is, in Schutz's terms, of 'primary relevance' because it is part of that 'sector of the world within which our projects can be materialized' (1946: 468).

Regina experienced a more abrupt change in her thinking. Like Colin, she
grew up knowing there was a family history of HD. Her father had onset in
his 30s and her brother learned (through linkage testing) that he was at
increased risk. HD was not, however, something that Regina dwelled on. She
wasn't 'hiding from it', she just hadn't made up her mind. As she explained:

I was riding the fence. I never decided whether I wanted it done or didn't
decide that I didn't want it done. I was sittin' on the fence.

After her father died, things changed. Regina was, nonetheless, at a loss to
explain why she suddenly felt that it was time to decide about predictive
testing.

I don't know why it's changed. I don't know whether it's cos my life's been so busy for such a long time that I never had time to think about it, because Dad was so sick and everything else. . . . or that my life has finally come down enough, has slowed me down enough that I've finally had time to think about it . . . but all of a sudden it was bugging me all the time, and I wasn't sleeping and, not being a real religious person, I thought 'somebody somewhere is telling me that it's time I made the decision in my life.' So I figured like . . . it wouldn't be in the forefront so much, like I don't mean forefront in the sense of always talking about it but (pause), instead of being in the subconscious it was consciously there all the time. I thought for something that's never bugged me before there's got to be a reason for it so I just made the phone call and did it.

### 'Things I add up in my head'

Regina isolates a moment of change in which she realises that risk is 'consciously there all the time'. Such moments signal a transition between two contiguous modes of cognition. The 'monothetic' mode of cognition arises from the world of routine activities and taken-for-granted understandings which structure lay actors' commonsense knowledge while the 'polythetic' mode of cognition involves the world of considered alternatives and the rational weighing of costs and benefits that typifies calculative action (Bloor 1995). These two modes are not discrete: indeed, it is the act of shifting between habitual and calculative modes of cognition that brings a particular topic into or out of focus, placing it at the centre or periphery of attention and subjecting it to a greater or lesser degree of consideration (Schutz 1970).

Many study participants compartmentalised and therefore sustained a distinction between their taken-for-granted understandings of risk and a more objectified (though not always scientific) knowledge of risk. How risk felt differed from how abstract reason suggested it ought to feel. How risk felt did, however, also become the object of consideration. Thus, it too became incorporated into the social and biographical calculus of risk. This calculus transformed an abstract knowledge of patterns of inheritance and the typical age of onset into something infinitely more complex than any Mendelian calculus of a priori risk.

The transformation is striking in Helen's account because she so clearly interleaves her own biography and kinship relations with an understanding of Mendelian inheritance in order to render an abstract knowledge of risk subjectively meaningful. (As the reader will wish to know, Helen's mother's died of cancer at age 67.)

My risk is one in four but I consider it to be much less . . . The doctor made a point of saying it is one in four, that it doesn't matter how old your mother was if she wasn't confirmed as not having it then you are one in four . . . Although when I speak of it as one in four, mentally it's not . . . I couldn't put a figure on it, one in twenty, whatever, quite a bit less because of my mother's age and because I've never seen or been exposed to it. It's still something that is really foreign to me as much as I know that it shouldn't be. It's something that they have over there (in Britain) that doesn't come over here . . . I don't know that side of the family . . . Also, I figure the fact that I am that much older is a good sign. We'll give that another two or three percentage points, you know, all these little things that I add up in my head.

Helen's husband Duane was reassured to learn that Helen was not 'a real 50 : 50'. Referring to her risk as 'marginal', he said:

. . .there's a niggling doubt . . . but trying to be scientific about it, strictly scientific and not emotional kind of thing, I think it's almost as close to guaranteed negative as you can get.

Others were more reticent about speaking in such certain terms, especially when the test results were imminent. Albert had been through linkage testing and received a decreased risk. Elaborating on how he kept himself alert to the possibility that the direct test could reveal that he had inherited the mutation associated with HD, Albert described a strategy he used to prevent himself from taking things for granted:

I figured well, gee whiz, if I had a two percent probability for HIV how would I feel? [pause] Devastated . . . It (two per cent) was still a significant amount.

Regina, on the other hand, minimised the potential impact of her test results but held open the possibility there might be some inchoate system of hereditary justice:

Say I knew I was going to be the lucky one, once I know I'm either going to let out a huge sigh of relief or [lengthy pause] I just keep telling myself that it hasn't missed a generation in a really long time in our family, as far back as I know it hasn't missed a generation and I figure I'm due.

Nigel also suggested there is some sort of HD scoreboard which must eventually tally. Though this conflicts with Mendelian assumptions about the random nature of gene transmission, Nigel clearly understands that he and his siblings each have a separate 50 : 50 chance of having inherited the mutation. It is just that pure chance does not help him to make sense of risk:

Okay, let's step up to the plate here. We're batting a 1,000 per cent you know, my grandmother had it, my aunt had it, my Dad now has it, someone's gotta to break this cycle. The odds are in my favour. Plus I was thinking that if I can break this cycle I could definitely give my brother and sister some confidence that, you know, well Nigel doesn't have it or, if I do have it, they've got a 50 : 50 chance just like I had and if I do have it then that's four with it and none without it, so they've got a good chance of breaking that themselves.

Nigel hopes to 'break the cycle' or at least give his siblings the feeling that they have a 'good chance'. This is possible no matter what the outcome of Nigel's test because (in keeping with his baseball analogy) he has covered all the bases. If he does not have the gene, it will give his siblings confidence. If he does have the gene, they will still have the same 50 per cent chance he had; moreover, the score will be four with and none without it so their 'odds' will have improved.

Other test candidates looked for a sign indicating the probable outcome of predictive testing. When Anne's doctor asked about her 'gut feeling', Anne said she thought she 'had it'. Elaborating on why, Anne said:

I see so much of my Dad in me, so many little physical things, more than my brother. My brother seems to be more like my mother's side of the family . . . Like my Dad had this circulation problem and . . . I have it and it's to do with your hands. They just get frozen all the time . . . When I would hold hands with him I could feel his hands, or often if I hold hands with myself if I'm sitting with my hands on my lap that's the feeling I used to have when my father used to hold my hand. It's just sort of an eerie feeling of knowing.

Just before her test results, Anne vacillated between thinking she knew what her results would be and feeling as if her thinking could itself have an impact on the results.

I was thinking 'show me a sign, give me a sign it's gonna be yes or it's gonna be no.' And I went for this long walk down where I always walk . . . and they have all the railroad cars down there and I kept seeing Xs. Wherever I looked there seemed to be Xs and I thought 'good that's negative, X is a negative thing, that's mean it's not gonna happen, I'm not going to have it.' I was convinced that day I didn't have it. And then another day I went along and I saw all these Ys and I though 'oh oh, that means yes.' But I was trying to talk myself into not having it and I thought well that can't happen because it's already happened. Whatever happened has happened. I've just got to confront it. And then you keep thinking why am I doing this? why am I being tested [sigh]?

Anne did not comment on the symbolism of the Xs and Ys (although she may have been thinking of sex chromosomes and the possibility of inheriting HD from her father) but she did come to a startling realisation—that is, 'whatever happened *has* happened'.

Though it seems obvious, the test has no bearing on whether an at-risk individual will eventually develop HD. The dice has already been cast. This logic is not, however, the only lived logic of predictive testing; from the standpoint of the test candidate awaiting results, it feels as if the act of taking the test is equivalent to throwing the dice. Predictive testing is confusing precisely because it is as if the act of coming to know one's genetic status is what determines one's genetic status. Of course this cannot be: as Anne says, 'it can't happen because it's already happened' yet, in another sense, it has not yet happened. This paradox is aptly described as the 'interpenetration of two mutually exclusive tenses' (Massumi, cited in Carter 1995: 136).

### 'This thing inside me'

When does an hereditary disease 'begin'? At the moment of conception? With the knowledge that one has inherited the mutation? Once symptoms are undeniable? With diagnosis?

Anne found there was quite a difference between thinking you have the mutation associated with HD and being told you have it. She recalled the moment when she and her husband learned her results in the following way:

> The doctor just showed me the paper and said . . . 'you have inherited Huntington's disease.' It was out on the table very quickly . . . And then I just froze. . . . I was holding Mark's hand and I just froze. . . . I didn't cry or anything . . . And I was fine that night, I was sort of numb. . . . and then (the next morning) I broke down. I came out of the shower and went to pieces. Had a good cry and got angry . . . And I think the thing I said is 'I just don't want this thing inside me. I don't want it.' I just didn't want that thing inside me . . .

The doctor assured Anne that she was not showing any symptoms of HD. Nonetheless, it was several months before Anne came to the conclusion that 'you can't worry about this thing waiting to happen, you got to get on with life.'

Regina also learned that she had inherited the mutation associated with HD. Matter of fact in her assessment of this news, Regina said:

> I'm still the same person, I just have this bit of information that other people don't have. It doesn't make me any different. And I guess that's what I've told myself is that knowing what I know, just sit back and think about it realistically, is it altering my life now? I say no. Is there anything I can't do? No. Well then why walk on egg shells?

For Regina, there was a certain utility in knowing that she had one little 'bit of information', one 'objective fixed point' on life's uncertain terrain (Bury 1982: 179). As she said, nothing has changed: 'It needn't be dealt with again until the time that it occurs in my life'.

Michael made a similar point. Reflecting on his observations of a support group for people who were 'gene positive', he said that most people were not 'down in the dumps'. He said there was, however, one woman who was there with her husband and they were not handling things very well. 'They're suffering the disease that she doesn't have yet, that's the kind of feeling I have.'

Rothman suggests that it is 'in the nature of this growing world of genetic prediction that we offer information "out of time", abruptly and without context of lived experience.' Illness no longer comes "in a context, in the course of a life, unfolding itself over time' (1996: 32). It comes before its time. As Peter said:

> It's an odd thing isn't it to tell somebody immanently you're going to get this? . . . People have the choice and some people think they're strong enough to know the answer and may not be.

Peter's wife Marie learned that she had inherited the mutation. Peter did not think she was handling it well; he said she had a certain 'rigidity' and that she was very closed about her feelings.

Colin also found predictive testing a bit 'scary'. When he and his wife learned that he did not inherit the genetic mutation associated with HD, the overwhelming feeling was, however, anti-climactic.

> When I got the results I was not ready, it just went right over my head. It didn't fizzle me at all . . . we had convinced ourselves that I had the gene and probably already had the disease . . . I guess we wanted to make sure that we wouldn't have this big let down . . . Unfortunately I think we did have a let down. The let down was that this thing that I've been carrying on my back for about 24 years, knowing my risk, has been such a big part of me that I just can't throw it off my shoulder and walk out and do a few cartwheels.

Risk was a part of Colin's self-identity. Moreover, he also experienced survivor's guilt, a concept that he had read about in the literature. He couldn't tell his older brother (who had been diagnosed with HD) that he had not inherited the mutation though he was able to spend more time with his brother without feeling as if he were looking at himself several years down the road. As Colin said, 'I don't have that fear any more. That's when you feel like your load's lightened.'

Helen had a more immediate emotional response to learning that she had not inherited the mutation. She was 'insanely calm' before the news and, then 'really vile' afterwards. Her husband Duane advised that it would be a good idea to 'sort of brace the partner that something like that might happen'. He was caught off guard by what he called a 'negative negative' . . . 'she was out of control'. Within a few weeks, however, the whole experience began to fade. As Helen said:

. . . [once] I was over the initial week or two of shock, it's almost like I dreamed it, like it didn't happen, it's in the past. It feels more like a bad dream now and I have to remind myself it actually did happen.

Things were less straightforward for Gabriella and her family:

The geneticist told me how many repeats I had.[9] Then he said 'we don't usually tell people how many repeats they have but we're telling you that you have 36 repeats because you're in this odd category of people'.

Gabriella had an intermediate allele and it was uncertain whether she would eventually develop HD. Her son Jason was annoyed with all the questions everyone asked. He initially interpreted the results in a very straightforward way: 'Mum has the gene'. Reflecting on what this meant to him, he then said:

It becomes one of the things that is in my family and one of the effects is that you have this news that you can tell people . . . I don't like the term but our family has this affliction. Whereas before it was just a sort of nebulous concept, maybe now it's a bit more concrete.

Later in the interview, Jason was less certain about how to frame his mother's test results. He recalled trying to explain what they meant to an old girlfriend who reacted as if he and his family 'ought to have succumbed to natural selection or something.' The experience convinced him that there are problems with how we think and talk about hereditary risk. As he explained:

We all have the Huntington's gene . . . we just have different forms . . . I started talking about it differently to a large degree because my Mum has the intermediate form. It then becomes important because if she has 40 repeats, if that was the number . . . they would say 'no you don't have the gene.' Well you've got pretty well all the same bits of DNA, you're just missing a CAG repeat and that changes the complete nature of that gene? I think people would agree that it doesn't. You still have basically the same thing it's just slightly different. So that might help. I don't know . . . It's a much harder thing to explain. We like things that are final, like you have it or you don't.

Jason raises a fundamental problem: shorthand ways of speaking about having or not having 'the gene for HD' oversimplify the genetics as well as the lived experience of HD and predictive testing. There is, as Jason points out, a need to articulate some form of alternative discourse on the meaning and significance of hereditary risk.

## Conclusion

Theories of Mendelian inheritance frame risk in static, objective terms. They abstract hereditary risk from the messiness of human contingency and biography; they separate self from the risk of disease and assume randomness and pure chance. They provide a framework for calculating the odds of inheriting a disorder but they do not recognise the livable framework or 'habitus' (Bourdieu 1977) for understanding risk as it emerges within everyday life.

Though lay constructions of risk appear to contradict the theories of Mendelian genetics, they offer a coherent framework for understanding the habitual as well as explicitly considered realities of hereditary risk and its modification through predictive testing. Factors such as geographic and social proximity to an affected family member are as important as biological ties in explaining test candidates and their families' intersubjective constructions of hereditary risk. Abstracted from an awareness of the familial interactions which shape the everyday experience of risk, such logic may appear ill-founded. Nonetheless, it is precisely this type of complex social, rather than biological, calculation which shapes everyday understandings and experiences of hereditary risk.

Adapting and modifying the framework of Mendelian inheritance, test candidates and their families jointly engage in a complex social calculus of risk. This calculus is fluid and contingent rather than static, intersubjective rather than objective, and creative yet coherent. Further, as many family members as well as test candidates suggest, lay understandings of risk are also recursive: it is problematic to attend too closely (or not closely enough) to risk. Indeed, the ability to offer a metacommentary on what can and cannot be taken for granted is, in and of itself, an intriguing feature of lay risk that warrants more extensive treatment than we can offer here.

Existing studies on predictive testing have for the most part focused on the psychosocial and clinical implications of receiving an informative test result. The 'world of routine activities' (Schutz 1967) has, therefore, been neglected. If, however, the flux of risk is shaped by the way in which biography and the life trajectory unfold (McKellin et al. 1995), there is good reason to attend more closely to lay actors' habitual as well as rational understandings of hereditary risk. Though we have, in this chapter, examined lay constructions of risk solely within the context of predictive testing for HD, we suspect that our findings will have significant implications for sociological research on a range of other heritable conditions. Even with its comparatively straightforward genetics, HD creates the possibility for highly nuanced yet diverse interpretations of hereditary risk. These interpretations stretch our culturally-available frameworks revealing much about the shortcomings of viewing hereditary risk through the lens of a predominantly rational discourse.

## Acknowledgements

This research was carried out in collaboration with the Huntington Disease Predictive Testing Research Group at the University of British Columbia in Vancouver, Canada. We especially wish to thank Dr. Michael Hayden, members of the clinical and research team, and the study participants without whom there would be no such research. The research was also supported by grants to William McKellin from the Medical Services Foundation of British Columbia, the University of British Columbia Hampton Fund and the Huntington Society of Canada. In addition, Susan Cox received a Doctoral Fellowship from the Social Sciences and Humanities Research Council of Canada. An earlier and shorter version of this chapter was presented at the 1998 International Sociological Association Meetings in Montréal.

## Notes

1  Proband is the term used in clinical genetics to designate the index person or first contact for a family with a history of an hereditary condition.

2  Mendelian theories of inheritance are based on a foundation of transmission genetics established by Mendel in 1865 and rediscovered in the early 20th century. Through his classic experiments with pea plants, Mendel realised there are paired units of inheritance (*i.e.* genes): these units are discrete and where one such unit (or allele) is recessive and the other dominant, the recessive allele retains its identity and may be expressed in a subsequent generation (*i.e.* when two recessive alleles are paired together). Mendelian genetics also asserts the randomness of inheritance such that alleles at different genetic loci are distributed independently during meiosis (McConkey 1993).

3  The degree of expansion in this region is, at its upper limits positively correlated with earlier age of onset for HD but, given the wide variance in the correlation for most repeat ranges, these data are only considered useful in a small number of classes (Duyao *et al.* 1993, Simpson *et al.* 1993).

4  Gender differentials in uptake for predictive testing remain an underanalysed phenomenon. Bloch *et al.* (1989: 222) suggest that women's more intimate involvement with reproduction and child-rearing, coupled with 'the apparently greater capacity of men to deny their feelings and avoid looking at the painful implications of their situation', may help to explain the differential representation of women and men. In addition, it may be that the phenomenon simply reflects the fact that women do, overall, make use of the health care system with much greater frequency than do men.

5  Many at-risk individuals wait until they are past the typical age of onset before requesting predictive testing. Hence there is a decreased chance of learning that they have the gene for HD (Bloch *et al.* 1989).

6  Pseudonyms are used here and some details were omitted to preserve anonymity.

7  Duchenne is a sex-linked hereditary disorder that manifests itself in males but is transmitted by females. It is a muscle-wasting disease that occurs in childhood causing progressive deterioration and death in late adolescence (Parsons and Atkinson 1992).

8   Maggie's father had not been diagnosed with HD, thus Maggie and her siblings were at 25 per cent a priori risk. Her brother's diagnosis confirmed that their father must have been a gene carrier and thus Maggie's a priori risk increased to 50 per cent.
9   Given concerns about how people would interpret the implications of this information for age of onset, there has been considerable debate about whether or not repeat numbers should be provided to test candidates (Burgess and Hayden 1996). At the time of this study, most test candidates were not given their repeat number.

## References

Benjamin, C.M., Adam, S., Wiggins, S., Theilmann, J.L., Copley, T.T. and Bloch, M. (1994) Proceed with care: direct predictive testing for Huntington Disease, *American Journal of Human Genetics*, 55, 606–17.

Berger, P. and Luckmann, T. (1966) *The Social Construction of Reality: a Treatise in the Sociology of Knowledge*. New York: Penguin Press.

Bloch, M., Fahy, M., Fox, S. and Hayden, M. (1989) Predictive testing for Huntington's Disease: 11 demographic characteristics, life style patterns, attitudes and psychological assessments of the first fifty-one test candidates, *American Journal of Medical Genetics*, 217–224.

Bloch, M., Adam, S., Fuller, A., Kremer, B., Welsh, J.P. and Wiggins, S. (1993) Diagnosis of Huntington Disease: a model for the stages of psychological response based on experience of a predictive testing program, *American Journal of Medical Genetics*, 368–74.

Bloor, M. (1995) A user's guide to contrasting theories of HIV-related risk behaviour. In Gabe, J. (ed) *Medicine, Health and Risk: Sociological Approaches*. Oxford; Blackwell Publishers.

Bourdieu, P. (1977) *Outline of a Theory of Practice*. Cambridge: Cambridge University Press.

Boutté, M.I. (1988) Genetic prophecy: the promises and perils of the new technology. Paper presented at the American Anthropological Association Conference, Phoenix, AZ.

Brandt, J., Quaid, K., Folstein, S., Gerber, P., Malstri, N. and Abbott, M. (1989) Presymptomatic diagnosis of delayed-onset disease with linked DNA markers: the experience of Huntington's Disease, *Journal of the American Medical Association*, 261, 3108–14.

Brinkman, R.R., Mezei, M.M., Theilmann, J., Almqvist, E. and Hayden, M. (1997) The likelihood of being affected with Huntington Disease by a particular age, for a specific repeat size, *American Journal of Human Genetics*, 60, 1202–10.

Burgess, M.M. (submitted) Contextual bioethics: everyday morality in genetic testing.

Burgess, M.M. and Hayden, M.R. (1996) Patients' rights to laboratory data: trinucleotide repeat length in Huntington Disease, *American Journal of Medical Genetics*, 62, 6–9.

Bury, M. (1982) Chronic illness as biographical disruption, *Sociology of Health and Illness*, 4, 167–82.

Carter, S. (1995) Boundaries of danger and uncertainty: an analysis of the technological culture of risk assessment. In Gabe, J. (ed) *Medicine, Health and Risk: Sociological Approaches*. Oxford: Blackwell Publishers.

Conrad, P. (1990) Qualitative research on chronic illness: a commentary on method and conceptual development, *Social Science and Medicine*, 30, 1257–63.

Cox, S.M. (1998) Managing to communicate: Family talk about genetic risk and Huntington Disease. Paper presented at the Qualitative Health Research Conference, Vancouver, British Columbia.

Cox, S.M. (in progress) *'It's Not a Secret But . . .' Predictive Testing and Patterns of Communication about Genetic Information in Families At Risk for Huntington Disease*. Unpublished Doctoral Dissertation. University of British Columbia.

Duyao, M., Ambrose, C., Myers, R., Novelletto, A., Persichettit, F., Frontali, M., *et al.* (1993) Trinucleotide repeat length instability and age of onset in Huntington's Disease, *Nature Genetics*, 4, 387–92.

Fox, S., Bloch, M., Fahy, M. and Hayden, M.R. (1989) Predictive testing for Huntington Disease: I Description of a pilot project in British Columbia, *American Journal of Medical Genetics*, 211–16.

Frank, A.W. (1991) *At the Will of the Body: Reflections on Illness*. Boston: Houghton Mifflin Company.

Gifford, S. (1986) The meaning of lumps: a case study of the ambiguities of risk. In Janes, C., Stall, R. and Gifford, S. (eds) *Anthropology and Epidemiology: Interdisciplinary approaches to the Study of Health and Diseases*. Boston: Reidel.

Goldberg, Y.P., Rommens, J.M., Andrew, S.E., Hutchinson, G.B., Lin, B. and Theilmann, J., (1993) Identification of an Alu retrotransposition event in close proximity to a strong candidate gene for Huntington's Disease, *Nature*, 362, 370–3.

Green, J., Richards, M., Murton, F., Statham, H. and Hallowell, N. (1997) Family communication and genetic counselling: the case of hereditary breast and ovarian cancer, *Journal of Genetic Counselling*, 6, 45–60.

Hayden, M. (1981) *Huntington's Chorea*. Berlin: Springer-Verlag.

Hayden, M.R. (1994) Huntington's Disease: Diagnosis, treatment and current research. Keynote address, Huntington Society of Canada Conference for Families, Vancouver, British Columbia.

Hayes, C. (1992) Genetic testing for Huntington's Disease—a family issue, *New England Journal of Medicine*, 327, 1449–51.

Huntington, G. (1967 [1872]) On Chorea, *Archives of Neurology*, 17, 33–5.

Huntington Society of Canada (1996) Understanding Huntington's Disease: a resource for families. Huntington Society of Canada: Cambridge, Ontario.

Huntington's Disease Collaborative Research Group (1993) A novel gene containing a trinucleotide repeat that is expanded and unstable on Huntington's Disease chromosomes, *Cell*, 72, 971–83.

Kavanagh, A.M. and Broom, D.H. (1998) Embodied risk: my body, myself? *Social Science and Medicine*, 46, 437–44.

Kessler, S. (1993) Forgotten person in the Huntington Disease family, *American Journal of Medical Genetics*, 48, 145–50.

Kessler, S. and Bloch, M. (1989) Social system responses to Huntington Disease, *Family Process*, 59–68.

Lakoff, G. and Johnson, M. (1980) *Metaphors We Live By*. Chicago: University of Chicago Press.

Lee, R.M. (1993) *Doing Research on Sensitive Topics*. London: Sage Publications.

Lippman-Hand, A. and Fraser, F.C. (1979) Genetic counselling—the postcounseling period: parent's perceptions of uncertainty, *American Journal of Medical Genetics*, 4, 51–71.

McConkey, E.H. (1993) *Human Genetics: The Molecular Revolution*. Boston: Jones and Bartlett Publishers.

McKellin, W., Cox, S.M. and Burgess, M.M. (1995) Varieties of genetic experience: patient and family members' understanding of medical genetic testing for single and multi-factor conditions: Huntington Disease, Alzheimer Disease, and familial breast cancer. Paper presented at the American Anthropological Association, Washington, D.C.

Mishler, E.G. (1991) *Research Interviewing: Context and Narrative*. Cambridge: Harvard University Press.

Nelkin, D. and Lindee, M.S. (1995) *The DNA Mystique: the Gene as a Cultural Icon*. New York: W.H. Freeman and Company.

Nukaga, Y. and Cambrosio, A. (1997) Medical pedigrees and the visual production of family disease in Canadian and Japanese genetic counselling practice. In Elston, M.A. (ed) *The Sociology of Medical Science and Technology*. Oxford: Blackwell Publishers.

Parsons, E. and Atkinson, P. (1992) Lay constructions of genetic risk, *Sociology of Health and Illness*, 14, 437–55.

Press, N. and Browner, C.H. (1997) Why women say yes to prenatal diagnosis, *Social Science and Medicine*, 45, 979–89.

Rapp, R. (1988) Chromosomes and communication: the discourse of genetic counselling, *Medical Anthropology Quarterly*, 2, 143–57.

Reddy, M.J. (1993) The conduit metaphor—a case of frame conflict in our language about language. In Ortony, A. (ed) *Metaphor and Thought*. (2nd Edition). Cambridge: Cambridge University Press.

Richards, L. (1994) User's mistake as developer's challenge: designing the new NUD*IST, *Qualitative Health Research*, 3.

Richards, M. (1993) The new genetics: some issues for social scientists, *Sociology of Health and Illness*, 15, 567–86.

Richards, M. (1996) Families, kinship and genetics. In Marteau, T. and Richards, M. (eds) *The Troubled Helix: Social and Psychological Implications of the New Human Genetics*. Cambridge: Cambridge University Press.

Richards, M. and Ponder, M. (1996) Lay understanding of genetics: a test of a hypothesis, *Journal of Medical Genetics*, 33, 1032–6.

Richards, T.J. and Richards, L. (1994) Using computers in qualitative research. In Denzin, N.K. and Lincoln, Y.S. (eds) *Handbook of Qualitative Research*. Thousand Oaks, CA: Sage Publications.

Rothman, B.K. (1996) Medical sociology confronts the genome, *Medical Sociology News: a Newsletter of the BSA*, 22, 23–35.

Schneider, D.M. (1980) *American Kinship: a Cultural Account*. Chicago: University of Chicago Press.

Schutz, A. (1946) The well-informed citizen: an essay on the social distribution of knowledge, *Social Research*, 13, 463–78.

Schutz, A. (1967) *Phenomenology of the Social World*. Evanston, Illinois: Northwestern University Press.

Schutz, A. (1970) *Reflections on the Problem of Relevance*, (ed) Zaner, R. New Haven: Yale University Press.

Shakespeare, J. (1992) Communication in Huntington's Disease families. Paper presented at the Third European Meeting on Psychosocial Aspects of Genetics, University of Nottingham.

Smith, D. (1987) *The Everyday World as Problematic: a Feminist Sociology.* Toronto: University of Toronto Press.

Wexler, A. (1995) *Mapping Fate: a Memoir of Family, Risk, and Genetic Research.* New York: Times Books.

Wexler, N.S. (1979) Russian roulette: the experience of being at risk for Huntington's Disease: harbinger of the new genetics. In Kessler, S. (ed) *Genetic Counselling: Psychological Dimensions.* New York: Academic Press.

Yoxen, E.J. (1982) Constructing genetic diseases. In Wright, P. and Treacher, A. (eds) *The Problem of Medical Knowledge: Examining the Social Construction of Medicine.* Edinburgh: Edinburgh University Press.

# III: The Social Impact and Implications of Genetics

# Defining the 'social': towards an understanding of scientific and medical discourses on the social aspects of the new human genetics

*Sarah Cunningham-Burley and Anne Kerr*

## Introduction

All of the people associated with the new human genetics, be they scientists, clinicians, counsellors, patients, commentators or critics, tend to agree that these developments have enormous social and ethical implications (House of Commons Science and Technology Select Committee 1995, Nuffield Council on Bioethics 1993). Consequently, there is considerable discussion about the social aspects of the new genetics in professional literatures, the popular media and other public settings. The way in which 'the social' is framed within these accounts is an important marker of the interests and relative power of the groups concerned with the new human genetics. Scientists and clinicians are powerful players in such discussions and seem to be able to direct attention towards the social *implications* of genetics, especially its beneficial applications. Where concerns are expressed, these tend to be narrowly focused on issues such as the commercialisation of genetic testing, or threats to individual autonomy. This limits more fundamental and critical discussion about the social values embedded in the knowledge and practices of the new human genetics itself.

Analysing how 'the social' is defined within these discourses, and understanding the interests that are served through particular rhetorical strategies, is of fundamental importance to sociologists wishing to engage critically with developments in the new genetics, and to contribute effectively to public debates and policy formation in this area. There is a need for an analysis of how scientific and medical discourses about the social aspects of the new genetics are constructed, employed and take effect. Identifying the dominant rhetoric in the area, alongside alternative discourses, opens the way towards further critical engagement with the new genetics. In this chapter we offer one such analysis, drawing on a range of writings about the social aspects of the new human genetics from within science, medicine and public health.

Our starting point is the now commonplace recognition that the cognitive authority of science rests not on an essentialist distinction between objective science and other knowledge and practice, but on the outcome of complex negotiations, and the interplay of a range of professionals' interests (Abbott

1988). The field of the new genetics has attracted commentary from many professional groups: scientists; clinicians; bioethicists; social scientists; and disability activists. It is in this context that scientists and clinicians involved in the new genetics are negotiating their position and professional status.

One way in which scientists protect their cognitive authority is through erecting rhetorical boundaries between science and society (Gieryn 1983, 1999). They promote a distinction between science and non-science in order to preserve their privileged status as experts about the natural world (Hilgartner 1990). This can involve them in drawing distinctions between legitimate and illegitimate training, methodology, topics and professional standards (Gieryn 1999). Often scientists distance themselves from other experts (including sociologists) but they can also debate the legitimacy of different types of science. Invariably their boundaries are based upon distinctions between science and society, including distinctions between the social and the natural realms, objectivity and subjectivity, and expertise and lay knowledge.

These boundaries are often found in scientific controversies, or when scientists make representations to public bodies, such as government committees (Gieryn 1999). However, we can also find them in scientists' discussions about the social aspects of their science in their professional journals. In the case of the new human genetics, scientists and clinicians write about the social aspects of the new genetics in a range of scientific, medical, ethical and social scientific professional journals aimed at different audiences. A study of these accounts is one route to understanding how they preserve their cognitive authority both to study genetics and to advise on its social consequences. Through studying these accounts, we can understand how scientists demarcate good science from bad; and scientific knowledge from its use and or abuse, thereby constructing and maintaining the boundary between science and society. We can then begin to renegotiation and challenge this boundary.

In this chapter we begin to unpack three important aspects of scientists' and clinicians' written accounts of the social aspects of the new human genetics: the social uses and abuses of genetics; eugenics and genetic determinism and professional responsibilities and expertise. We discuss how they treat the relationship between science and its application; scientific knowledge and social values; and scientists' role in the professional and public spheres. After providing some background context we identify the dominant and alternative discourses in each, and consider the different professional interests which they might represent. Inconsistencies and concerns within scientists' and clinicians' accounts are identified, and we argue that these can be usefully combined with social scientific analyses and commentaries in order to facilitate more reflexive, pluralistic and inclusive dialogue and decision making about the new human genetics.

## The study

Our orientation is predominantly British as we are currently engaged in research and debates in this context.[1] We therefore focus on the accounts of clinical and molecular geneticists as opposed to genetic counsellors (who are a key professional group in the USA), and contrast these with the accounts of public health specialists. Geneticists are of course central to decision-making and discussions about the new human genetics, whereas the latter are more peripheral. However, the new genetics has particular implications for epidemiology and preventative medicine, as well as public health's wider interest in the social aspects of health and disease. Although the literature in this area is so vast that we cannot offer complete bibliographic coverage, we have endeavoured to cover a range of journals and other texts, such as edited collections. Our aim has been to ensure wide coverage, in order to minimise the risk of selecting only those articles most frequently cited, and of promoting a hegemonic view of science; discourse is likely to be much more diverse. We have also tried to access accounts aimed at both specialised and more general audiences. Given the 'cross-over' between the social and biomedical sciences in this area we have reviewed a selection of social science, natural science and medical journals. Although these are mainly from a British perspective, we recognise that the nature of scientific and medical research means that an international (particularly North American) perspective is also important. This is recognised in some of the articles we reviewed.

We systematically considered articles about the social aspects of the new human genetics written by scientists, clinicians, and public health professionals from 1987–1997 in *Social Science and Medicine*, *Sociology of Health and Illness*, *American Journal of Public Health*, *British Journal of General Practice*, *British Journal of Obstetrics and Gynaecology*, and the *Journal of Medical Ethics*. This is supplemented with a selection of appropriate articles from a range of other publications—for example the *British Medical Journal*, *Lancet*, *New England Journal of Medicine*, *Journal of the American Medical Association*, *Nature*, *Science*, *American Journal of Human Genetics*, and the *Journal of Medical Genetics*—around key areas such as genetic screening, public involvement, and other social, legal and ethical issues. In total approximately 100 articles were reviewed, by one or other of the authors. Articles were analysed in terms of how the social context of the new genetics was addressed, and the contours which framed this conceptualisation.

Although such coverage cannot be viewed as comprehensive, it does provide an important resource for analysing scientists' and clinicians' accounts of the social aspects of the new human genetics. It complements our previous analyses of new genetics professionals' interview accounts (Kerr *et al.* 1997, 1998b) by giving us access to written material from a wider group of experts with an interest in this area. It also allows us to develop the more specific analysis of clinical accounts by authors such as Lippman (1992b) and to add further empirical flesh to the broader commentaries by authors such as Rose (1994) and Rothman (1998).

## Background to the new human genetics

A recognition of the troubled relationship between medicine, science, human genetics and eugenics must be the starting point for our analysis of contemporary scientists' and clinicians' accounts of the social aspects of the new human genetics (see Adams 1990, Kamrat-Lang 1995, Kerr *et al.* 1998b, Kevles 1986, Ludmerer 1989, MacKenzie 1981, Paul 1992, 1995 for detailed historical analyses). Its legacy means that those professionals working in this area have to acknowledge, at the very least, that science can be socially and politically driven or abused.

At its peak in the 1930s, eugenics had substantial support from the medical and scientific community and had a significant impact on medical and social services in the USA and Britain. However, developments in plant and animal genetics, empirical evidence which countered heredity theories and questioned the effectiveness of eugenic policies, increasing disquiet about sterilisation in the USA and elsewhere, and the atrocities of Nazi Germany, all contributed to a decline in human genetics after World War II. Population and experimental genetics diverged and the emerging discipline of clinical genetics distanced itself politically, socially and scientifically from its eugenic past. Keller has argued that this separation between physical traits and human behaviour gave genetics a new scientific respectability, based on its neutrality, and meant that it could develop unfettered by concerns about the relationship between nature and nurture, or science and society (Keller 1992).

The 1950s saw a rise in psychological and sociological explanations for human behaviour, and the optimistic development of a range of social and environmental interventions to improve the human condition. However, by the 1970s, as research in genetics was moving into the molecular era, genetic determinism was in vogue once more. Although eugenic laws were being repealed in North America and Scandinavia as late as the 1970s, sterilisation also continued in some institutions for the mentally ill under the cloak of voluntarism. The reinstatement of genetics as potentially beneficial, at least in the clinical setting, was beginning. Since then there has been an enormous popularisation of determinist science and powerful new alliances between universities, government and the biotechnology industry, culminating in the Human Genome Project (HGP). There is considerable bravado about the HGP's ability to produce the 'book of man' and cure genetic disease, the new social problem of our time. However, researchers in this field also frequently emphasise their balanced approach to genetics and the environment. They argue that earlier this century nature was inappropriately emphasised and in the 1950s nurture was reified, claiming that it is only now, as we move towards the end of the century, that both are recognised as important and intermeshed (Plomin and Craig 1997).

Scientific and technological developments have also meant that the clinical applications of genetic knowledge have become possible. Genetic testing and screening is currently available for serious clinical conditions in Britain and the USA, and research is also being conducted which could lead to the development of pre-symptomatic genetic testing for more common, and more complex diseases, as well as psychiatric disorders and behavioural traits. As Duster (1992) argues, although the 'front door' to eugenics appears to be closed, the 'back door' of disease prevention is now a reality.

The spectres of eugenics and genetic determinism, past and present, alongside the growing public scepticism about scientists' and doctors' authority (Beck 1992; Giddens 1991) have meant that today's scientists and clinicians must carefully negotiate the social and ethical implications of the new human genetics. Addressing 'the social' is therefore an important element of scientists' and clinicians' discourse, whether this is in the context of securing funds, engaging public support, or ensuring acceptable health care practice. However, engaging with social issues potentially undermines the cognitive authority of scientists by threatening the status of science as 'value free', and by challenging the important boundary between science and society.

Scientists address the relationship between science and society, more specifically between genetic knowledges, technologies, ideology and social issues, in various ways. The ways in which genetics can be used (for good or bad) and the role of scientists and clinicians in shaping or reflecting the values of society is a particular source of tension, and we focus firstly on these issues in the following analysis of published accounts. Secondly, eugenics and genetic determinism are especially thorny issues. These undermine the separation between knowledge and social values (or progress, in the case of eugenics), so dissociating them from the new human genetics is important for practitioners in this area. Thirdly, and more generally, the social and scientific responsibilities of scientists and clinicians and the extent of their expertise are important topics of discussion. The preservation of cognitive authority relies on scientists' successful management of the tension between interested concern and disinterested practice and on their adoption of appropriate professional and public roles at this interface. We now go on to investigate these issues in turn, starting with scientists' and clinicians' accounts of the social use and/or abuse of the new human genetics.

### Notes on scientific and clinical discourses

*The social uses and abuses of the new human genetics*
As Turney has noted, books about the Human Genome Project abound, and usually end with an obligatory chapter on its social, ethical and legal

implications (1993). However, these accounts invariably cast the science and technology of human genetics apart from their social and ethical context. Similarly, many of the accounts that we considered implicitly adopted this framework. For example, Tsui, writing on cystic fibrosis mutations in *Trends in Genetics*, concluded the article thus:

> the issues of population screening for CF carriers and prenatal testing must be considered at the social and ethical level before any broad scale program is implemented (1992: 398).

This repeated, if bland, recognition that there are social and ethical issues associated with the new human genetics formed the background to professionals' further acknowledgement of a limited set of social concerns. Two such issues were the threat to privacy and potential for discrimination (particularly in relation to insurance and employment); and the commercialisation of genetic testing. Clinical geneticists especially were wary of the unregulated development of genetic testing in the private sector (or reformed NHS in the UK) because this might not involve proper non-directive counselling. For example, Harper, a clinical geneticist working in Britain, wrote in the *British Medical Journal*, that where Huntington's disease was concerned,

> the most serious (problem) is the possibility of testing without giving information, counselling and support—especially worrying when economic pressure is being exerted to reduce health service costs and when some British laboratory services are being contracted out (Harper 1993: 397).

There was also concern about the provision of adequate and balanced information about tests to potential clients and the protection of their privacy and autonomy in decision-making (Mayeux and Schupf 1995, Sweeney 1997). This issue was especially acute because of the experiences associated with sickle cell carrier testing in the 1970s (Chapple 1992, Anionwu 1993), and the role of insurance in health care organisation, and the potential for discrimination (Billings *et al.* 1992b). There was also a focus on the specific issues relating to testing of children or new-borns (Clarke 1994a, Harper and Clarke 1995, Working Party of the Clinical Genetics Society (UK) 1994), and testing at a population-level (Clarke 1995, Harper 1992). These concerns suggest that some vocal clinical geneticists appeared to be especially keen to evaluate services before their full-scale provision; and to work together with psychologists and social scientists (Bekker *et al.* 1993; Marteau *et al.* 1994, Williamson *et al.* 1989). Discussions tended to concentrate on the social and ethical implications of genetic technologies for families and individuals (see Marteau and Richards 1996 for an extensive review). Occasionally some technical aspects of the science and technology came under scrutiny, particularly when the accuracy of testing was discussed (Johnston 1992; Almqvist *et al.* 1997).

More usually these accounts highlighted the potential benefits of genetic testing and stressed the increased amount of choice which genetic testing can give people about health care and its potential for alleviating suffering and disease. Part of this discourse involved appeals to gene therapies and treatments (Bell 1998), but prenatal genetic diagnosis was also lauded as a way of eliminating 'dreadful diseases' that 'plague human existence', or 'consumes the carriers identity' (Watson 1990; see also Shakespeare in this issue). An important feature of this discourse was the tendency to dissociate the elimination of disease from the elimination of people with the disease (Pembrey 1998, Wald *et al.* 1992, and see Sutton 1995). Overall, there was little reflection about the social aspects of disease definition and the social (as opposed to medical) problems of disability. However, some clinical geneticists, who deal directly with affected individuals and their families, were once again more circumspect. For example, Clarke argued, in a discussion about the Nuffield report on the ethics of genetic screening in the *Bulletin of Medical Ethics*, that Down's Syndrome is 'one way, among others, of being human' (Clarke 1994b: 19).

Much of the writing from a public health perspective continued this separation between science and its use/abuse in its focus on the potential or actual application of the new human genetics in public health programmes. Khoury *et al.* (1996), for example, explicitly distinguished the production of genetic science and technology from its use and or abuse, and therefore stressed the need for public health specialists to attend to concerns about autonomy, consent, confidentiality, privacy and education. Science was frequently portrayed as being progressive, and public health's contribution through epidemiological and evaluative studies was emphasised (Mayeux and Schupf 1995, Hiller *et al.* 1997, Holtzman 1997). For example, Mayeux and Schupf wrote:

New scientific and technical capabilities create new ethical, legal and social problems that affect both the medical community and the public health community . . . The rapid pace of scientific progress in molecular medicine suggests that all investigators concerned with public health questions should carefully consider the issues raised by this remarkable era of scientific progress (Mayeux 1995: 1283).

As with other scientists and clinicians, those writing from the public health perspective tended not to be critical of genetics per se, but rather of the introduction of screening programmes that had not been thoroughly tested, or which did not meet the criteria currently used in public health. For example, Stone and Stewart (1996) argued that the provision of information, which is often given as a justification for genetic screening, does not in itself encapsulate any preventive principle and does not therefore meet the established public health criteria for screening for disease. This challenged the assertion of the 'right to know' as justification for the application of genetic technologies in preventive health.

General statements about the social and ethical issues associated with the use and abuse of genetics deflect attention from the social influences on the production of scientific knowledge. Legitimate areas of 'social' concern in relation to the new genetics are also narrowly defined. This demarcates specific areas of concern, where professionals' expertise may help to safeguard the public. However, professionals were more attuned to stressing the benefits of their work which served as an implicit recognition of the importance of a social goal to their scientific endeavours.

*Eugenics and genetic determinism*
Although the atrocities of Nazi Germany were sometimes cited as a 'warning' to geneticists and society to be cautious and responsible (Board of Directors of the American Society of Human Genetics 1999, Watson 1990), in most of the work we have reviewed, scientists and clinicians allied to the new human genetics tended not to acknowledge eugenics or genetic determinism as legitimate concerns. The new genetics was characterised as a neutral scientific representation of bodily processes and its medically-based application was stressed, whereas eugenics tended to be characterised as a politically distorted pseudo-science, or abuse of genetics in the past (Galton and Galton 1998). New geneticists deployed historical, ethical and medical arguments to emphasise the importance of individual choice in contemporary medical genetics in contrast to the social control and population planning of the past (Ledly 1994), and were sometimes cautious about population level approaches (Harper 1992).

Despite this reluctance to address eugenics explicitly, its presence in popular consciousness and concerns about more recent examples of discrimination on biological grounds (for example sickle cell carrier screening, Chapple 1992, or in insurance, Low *et al.* 1998) did seem to mean that professionals tried not to overplay the importance of genetics in determining health or behaviour. Thus, although determinism is quite explicit amongst the popularisers of genetic science (for example Watson said of the HGP, 'a more important set of instruction books will never be found by humans' 1990: 44), there was concern in the accounts we reviewed that this might lead to unrealistic expectations of disease prevention on the part of the public (Gill and Richards 1998). Others cautioned against determinist language like 'the gene for . . .' (Billings *et al.* 1992a, Hubbard and Wald 1993), and some noted it might backfire on the profession. For example, Maddox, the editor of *Nature* wrote:

> Most geneticists will probably agree that nurture still has a place. But to fail to say as much, explicitly, may generate more disbelief and even resentment than ethical worries have yet engendered. That would be a misfortune for a programme of such high promise (1993: 107).

This tension around genetic determinism was particularly evident where behavioural genetics was concerned. Billings *et al.* (1992a), writing in *Social*

*Science and Medicine*, noted that the versions of the environment which can be studied by behaviour geneticists are very limited and that assumptions about environmental differences between twins raised apart weaken the quantitative geneticists case for heredity. Concerns about determinism and the complex links between genotype and phenotype were also raised (Alper and Beckwith 1993, Alper 1996a).

Those working in behavioural genetics such as Plomin *et al.* (1994) and Wiesel (1994) were, however, careful to stress the need for a balanced view of the relationship between nature and nurture. Bouchard also wrote:

> It [behavioural genetics] views humans as dynamic creative organisms for whom the opportunity to learn and to experience new environments amplifies the effects of the genotype on the phenotype (1994, 1701).

Similarly, the American Society of Human Genetics' (ASHG) statement on behavioural genetics emphasised its apolitical character and genes' influence on, rather than determination of, human behaviour (Sherman *et al.* 1997).

Within public health accounts there was also a tendency to avoid critical discussion about eugenics. Little consideration was given to the role of public health in the surveillance of the populations' health, despite the tension between public health's long time emphasis on the social causes of disease and the association between public health and eugenics earlier this century (Pernick 1997). Where concerns were expressed they tended to be subsumed within an optimistic outlook. For example, although Stone and Stewart (1996) were critical of genetic screening as currently conceptualised, they suggested further research and evaluation into its effects rather than its abandonment. Nevertheless, there was a critical element to the public health discourse about the new human genetics. For example, Lippman (1992a and b) criticised reductionism and determinism, which she argued are inherent in genetic approaches to human health, and McDermott (1998) has criticised biological determinism in genetic epidemiology.

The avoidance of direct discussion of eugenics suggests boundaries between past and present practice, and between bad, pseudo-science and good, socially useful science. This effectively deflects criticism and concern about eugenics in relation to contemporary genetics. However, some accounts were more critical, as professionals carefully managed issues of genetic determinism and the controversial area of behavioural genetics. Interestingly, separations were made between behavioural versus medical genetics on the basis of their subjectivity versus objectivity and/or their social (behavioural) versus medical (biological) subject matter. On the other hand, other more critical scientists' and clinicians' concerns about the values embedded in testing programmes blurred the boundary between the scientific and the social.

*Responsibility and expertise*

The importance of caution and wise judgements (Schmidtke 1994, Sweeney 1997) were frequently emphasised in the accounts that we reviewed. For example, Gill and Richards writing in the *British Medical Journal* state that 'those engaged in genetic research have a responsibility to draw attention to the limits as well as the potential of their findings' (1998: 570). Some scientists and clinicians also described their work as being guided by scientific curiosity and a desire to ameliorate the effects of disease (Beaudet 1998, Savill 1997a, Wilmut 1998).

It was also argued in places that scientists had to engage with social issues (Harper and Clark 1997), to work with society in the application of beneficial knowledge (Cantor 1990), and to prevent the abuse of genetic knowledge especially through open debate (*e.g.* in the Nuffield Report, 1993). Where concrete recommendations were mentioned these usually took the form of guidelines on clinical practice—for example testing children (Working Party of the Clinical Genetics Society 1994). Clinical geneticists were also more concerned with concrete responsibilities, such as the need to advise their clients bout the implications for insurance or employment or participating in genetic testing. More generally, however, these appeals to responsibility tended not to be translated into concrete policy recommendations, or explicit descriptions of responsibilities in practice. Rather they were more usually manifest in vague concerns about alleviating public fear and ignorance. Although professionals also sometimes appealed to the responsibility of the whole of humanity to use scientific knowledge properly, they clearly also saw themselves as having an important role to play in both reassuring and guiding society. For example, Watson wrote, 'we must work to ensure that society learns to use the information only in beneficial ways . . .' (1990: 46). The American Society on Human Genetics' statement on Behavioural Genetics recommended the education of both public and press concerning the 'facts' about genetic differences and stated that scientists have an obligation to be involved in such education (Sherman *et al.* 1997). Relatedly, Chapple argued in an editorial that 'public education is a prerequisite to the widespread introduction of testing with truly informed consent' (1992: 487) in order to prevent stigma and discrimination.

A more critical perspective was evident in some calls for professional education as genetics moved into the clinic, especially the primary care setting (Savill 1997b, Kinmouth *et al.* 1998). Alper, for example, stressed the need to educate clinicians on the complexity of the genotype-phenotype relationship to stem genetic determinism (1996b). There was also some scepticism amongst some clinical geneticists about the claim that education would reduce stigmatisation of people with genetic conditions (for example, Clarke 1994b). It was even noted that better education might well reduce rather than increase the level of uptake of genetic tests (Clarke 1994b).

Public health specialists also tended to emphasise their professional expertise. For example, it was argued that they ought to play an important role in evaluative studies of clinical application of the new human genetics (Serra-Pratt *et al.* 1998). In other places public health specialists emphasised their expert knowledge about screening (Stone and Stewart 1996). The views of the public tended to be accorded importance because they could be used to improve existing services (Smith and Coyle 1995), not because they could be used to help decide what services ought to be developed in the first place. However, there was, on occasion, more explicit reference to the need for public participation in evaluating the application of genetic testing, a position which is potentially more radical than that of other scientists and clinicians associated with the new human genetics (Hiller *et al.* 1997).

In these accounts, scientists' and clinicians portray themselves as neutral, by separating science from its application, yet concerned, by embracing some responsibilities. Their expertise in matters social was defined through their role as educators of both publics and other professional groups. Social responsibility requires engagement with social issues, yet the authority for scientists to be involved in this arena rests on the value neutrality of their work. Operating with these boundaries, which at once separate and blur the distinction between science and society, involves scientists in both embracing and deflecting social concerns.

**Discussion**

The framing of 'the social' in terms of the implications of the new human genetics, the discussions about eugenics and genetic determinism, and the characterisation of professionals' responsibilities and expertise in these accounts, should not be regarded as a disinterested portrayal of difficult issues. Scientists' and clinicians' emphasis on the applications or implications of the new human genetics, not the science or technology per se, implies that genetic science and technology is value-free. Yet, the social benefits of the science and its applications tended to be emphasised in these accounts. The provision of greater reproductive choice, the alleviation of 'suffering' associated with serious disease, greater understanding of disease processes, and better therapeutic interventions, were all highlighted. Whilst this blurs the boundary between science and its social value, it also perpetuates a medical model of disease and disability (see Shakespeare, this issue), thereby reasserting the boundary between the biological (or natural) and the social aspects of disability.

At the same time as claiming neutrality, professionals remained obviously concerned about what they characterised as the abuse of genetic knowledge, and thus separated beneficial use from abuse of science. More manageable issues like privacy, discrimination, choice and evaluation took precedence in this literature over more fundamental and potentially divisive concerns about eugenics, genetic determinism, geneticisation and further medicalisation, thereby enhancing other boundaries between science and pseudo-science or abuse of science. These accounts also delineated the expertise and responsibilities of professionals. They emphasised their key role in education, in defining who needs to be educated, and about what, but they distanced themselves from what they portrayed as the potential abuses of their findings. This establishes a flexible boundary between science and society which allows scientists to strategically distance themselves from responsibility for the social consequences of their knowledge while actively taking a part in shaping these very processes (through their role on advisory panels, for example).

However, dissent and differences of opinion were also evident in these accounts. Specialists in particular fields sometimes asserted their expertise and authority by calling for the education of other professional groups, or a greater role in evaluation of research and services. On other occasions, problematic areas of the new genetics, particularly behavioural genetics, were criticised by clinical and other geneticists. This seemed to separate such work from mainstream, clinically relevant research, implying in some ways that the former is more socially biased, or 'social' as opposed to medical in its subject-matter. We also found what might be called two 'minority discourses': one expressed by a group of mainly British clinical geneticists with a particular interest in the practical resolution of social and ethical concerns, and another expressed by a looser grouping of mainly North American scientists and clinicians with a more radical perspective on the relationship between scientific knowledge and social values. This first group emphasised the need for cautious evaluation and focused on responsibilities in practice. Some clinical geneticists were also keen to dissociate genetics from moves towards population screening, or from behavioural genetics. The boundary around appropriate practice was tightly drawn, separating this from some of the more extravagant claims of others about the potential benefits of genetic research. The second group was concerned about some of the values that shape scientific knowledge and medical practice, particularly in behavioural genetics where they questioned its determinism and reductive methodologies. This shows how boundaries between good (neutral) and bad (socially biased) science may be drawn differently by different professional groups, thus opening the way for further debate.

Although the public health discourse framed social and ethical issues in a similar way to other scientists and clinicians, genetic testing and screening were favoured as part of public health's own preventive strategies. Those working in public health also seemed particularly keen to emphasise their expertise in the evaluation of screening programmes. However, criticisms were voiced about the rationale of screening and about inappropriate reductionism and determinism. It was also argued in places that genetics is but one aspect of disease and therefore its prevention, and the dangers of 'geneticisation' were warned against (Holtzman 1997, Lippman 1993, Petersen 1998). This follows from the strong interest of public health specialists in environmental or social determinants of ill health, which undermines genetic determinism (Willis 1998). The relationship between the new genetics and public health is very much contested ground. The new genetics challenges some aspects of the public health approach, yet reinforces others.

Boundaries are likely to be drawn and redrawn as the diverse professionals in this field engage further with these debates.

Overall, these accounts mirror the discursive strategies we have previously identified in the interview accounts of new genetics professionals (Kerr *et al.* 1997, 1998b), and echo the demarcations discussed by Gieryn (1983). Distinctions were drawn between scientific knowledge and its application; good science and bad; genetics and eugenics; and professional expertise and public ignorance. These discursive boundaries protect scientists' cognitive authority by delineating their expertise and responsible practice from illegitimate forms of knowledge and applications. However, there is clearly considerable flexibility about what constitutes legitimate/illegitimate knowledge, practice and professional roles relating to the new human genetics, as the minority discourses suggest. The tensions between scientists' neutrality and their social/advisory role; and between both their abrogation and claiming of responsibility for the effects of their work suggest that the discursive boundary between the scientific and social realms is flexible. Flexibility is also apparent when we consider the inconsistencies in and between particular accounts and the concerns and criticisms that were expressed in certain accounts. For example, those who are critical of population screening and behavioural genetics define these domains as outside the bounds of acceptable research and practice because of their eugenic associations, whereas others argue that they are progressive and/or value-free. This clearly highlights a tension around what constitutes neutrality and between the importance of neutrality on the one hand, and social progress or benefits on the other.

Despite the obvious potential of this flexibility or inconsistency to undermine professionals' arguments and boundaries, their considerable autonomy, powerful economic ties with industry and government, and the high media profile of some, all suggest that their cognitive authority remains intact. More cautious or sceptical professionals appear to be able to manage the tension in and between their professional and public roles, and express concerns without undermining the fundamental tenets of much genetic research and service provision. Indeed, the resolution of concerns about particular types of research or inappropriate technological developments often depended upon further research (including evaluation) or enhanced service provision, further extending the remit of science and the authority of scientists.

## Conclusion

To conclude, however, we suggest that this flexibility might also be used to challenge the very boundaries that the authors erected in these accounts. For example, scientists' and clinicians' emphasis on the separate nature of the social realm, in which their knowledges and technologies are applied, does not square with their social concerns about this area. Recognition of such concerns strongly suggests that there are social values embedded in their theories and practices. The minority discourse of some North American scientists and others concerned by behavioural genetics blurs other boundaries between good and bad science, balance and bias and disease and personhood. Public health specialists' concerns about the evaluation of testing may also militate against a population approach because evaluation may show that genetic tests are not as popular with publics or health care providers as professionals might first assume. Indeed, uptake for many testing programmes has not been as great as anticipated (Clayton *et al.* 1996, Quaid and Morril 1993). The concerns about professional education also challenge the separation of experts and lay people evident in the dominant discourse in these accounts.

The radical potential of professionals' own concerns and criticisms might be usefully allied to social investigations and analyses of the new human genetics, thus pointing the way to a more reflexive and critical perspective on the new human genetics, which deconstructs rather than reinforces boundaries. Although sociologists clearly have their own boundaries to draw with respect to sociological research and responsibilities, we also have a strong tradition of trying to dismantle the boundaries between experts and laity, and scientific knowledge and its social context. With respect to the new human genetics there is a growing number of critical analyses and studies on how professionals, patients, publics and the media perceive and represent the new human genetics (for example, Conrad and Weinberg 1996, Davison *et al.* 1994, Duster 1989, Marteau and Richards 1996, Nelkin and Tancredi 1989, Nelkin 1994, Nelkin and Lindee 1995, Parsons and Atkinson 1992, Richards 1993, Kerr *et al.* 1997, 1998b, Lippman 1992a and b, Rose 1994, Rothman 1998, Shakespeare 1995, see also Shakespeare this issue).

In the British context, much of the work focuses on the implications of the new genetics and the evaluation of existing services (for example Davison *et al.* 1994, Mateau and Richards 1996, Richards 1993). This highlights the complex relationship between clients and professionals and their different perspectives on genetic risk and disease (Marteau *et al.* 1989, 1993, Parsons and Atkinson 1992, Wertz and Reilly 1992). However, this can be used to challenge the separation of knowledge from its social context as conceptualised in the dominant discourse. Such research also challenges the notion of clinicians' neutrality. For example, Michie *et al.* (1997) have uncovered the persistence of directive counselling amongst obstetricians. Rues and Freimer (1997) have also reported that psychiatrists are much more likely to endorse termination for bipolar disorder than parents, support group members or medical students. This highlights the values implicit in genetic counselling and blurs the boundary between neutral knowledge and 'biased' application. It also problematises the boundary between choice and coercion on which the distinction between genetics and eugenics so often rests. Although there are still examples of an assumed 'deficit' in the public's understanding of genetics in the social scientific literature and a pre-occupation with education (Richards and Ponder 1996, Richards 1997, Sorenson and Cheuvront 1993), much of the social scientific work in this area takes lay perspectives seriously (Kerr *et al.* 1998a and c, Lambert and Rose 1996, Macintyre 1995). The demonstration of the ambivalence of the lay public towards carrier testing for cystic fibrosis has also had concrete effects in stemming the tide of genetic testing. Several community-based testing programmes, have not gone beyond the pilot stage because of lack of public enthusiasm (Bekker *et al.* 1993, Clayton 1996, Williamson *et al.* 1989).[2]

Social scientists with an interest in science and medicine could therefore form valuable alliances with critical scholars in the scientific, medical and public health disciplines to undermine the notions of value-free science and an ignorant public, to counter indifference towards eugenics, and to challenge the notion that 'biological disease' can be separated from the social world. For example, clinical geneticists' and social scientists' concerns about the practical context of genetic testing and counselling, particularly its value-laden character, could be developed into a more wide-ranging exploration of the values which shape genetic science and technology as a whole, not just in relation to the processes which shape application. This would also challenge the presupposed beneficence of the new human genetics and facilitate a more robust evaluation of its aims and values as well as its practical execution.

Social scientists could also work more closely with clinical geneticists in the evaluation of existing services, and try to involve the lay public in this process. Sociologists in particular could capitalise on the current interest in greater public involvement in evaluation of the new genetics, and promote a more thorough consideration of the lay public's areas of expertise (Kerr *et al.* 1998b and c). This would break down the traditional divide between scientific experts and others. We could also think creatively about how to democratise decision-making about genetic science and technology at all levels of research and application, not just at the stage of evaluation. This could involve forming other alliances with groups of the lay public with an interest in having their voices heard, and trying to find better ways of accessing the views of marginalised and oppressed groups of people so as to involve them in this process.

We are, of course, under no illusions about the powerful barriers to such a radical approach to the study of, and policy about, the new human genetics. The narrow remit of research funding, passive media coverage and the elitism of policy-making means that the more fundamental concerns about social context as opposed to social implications can be easily ignored or dismissed by people with the power to influence the quality of public discussion and decision-making. There are also many barriers to the boundary-crossing and deconstruction that we wish to encourage. Scientists and clinicians sympathetic to the sociological agenda must tread a fine line between critical involvement in and ostracism from their communities. Medical sociologists too must carefully negotiate the twin poles of biological and sociological essentialism. However, a recognition and detailed exploration of professional interests, and the rhetorical strategies which maintain them could, as Guston argues, 'improve the position of science in society, for society's ultimate benefit' (1999: 89). Many professionals within the new genetics and broader scientific and clinical communities are already cautious and reflective about their research and practices, and will therefore be more willing to enter into a dialogue with social scientists who are sceptical and critical of some genetic research and practice. Defining the social in relation to the new human genetics need not be a way of supporting the status quo if social scientists, radical scientists, practitioners and the lay public work together to expose and question the values and practices that it involves.

## Notes

1    We have recently completed a study *The Social and Cultural Impact of the New Genetics* (with Amanda Amos) funded by the ESRC under the Risk and Human Behaviour Programme, Grant Number L21125 2003. We are currently engaged in work analysing the discourses of a range of professional groups including bioethicists (SCB, AK), the social construction of cystic fibrosis (AK), the history of eugenics (AK with Tom Shakespeare), disability and the new genetics (SCB with Tom Shakespeare), and the intelligence debate (SCB, AK).

2    As with the dominant professional discourses outlined earlier, there are also more radical challenges from within social science, with commentators and researchers from a range of perspectives broadly including feminism, social constructionism and cultural studies (Asch and Geller 1996, Hartouni 1991, Heath 1998, Mahowald *et al.* 1996, Nelkin and Lindee 1995, Press and Brown 1994, Rapp 1998). Work carried out under the ELSI programme within the Human Genome Project, especially in its earlier phases, included both research which focused on the broader social issues, as well as the impacts of specific applications. Jeungst (1996) has argued that the programme is now narrower in its focus, thus curtailing the funding of work with more radical potential. No such equivalent ring fencing of money has taken place within the UK, although the Wellcome Trust has recently set up a Medicine in Society Programme to support research on the social, ethical and other consequences of developments in medicine and biology.

## References

Abbott, A. (1988) *The System of Progressions: an Essay on the Division of Expert Labour*. Chicago: The University of Chicago Press.
Adams, M.B. (eds) (1990) *The Wellborn Science: Eugenics in Germany, France, Brazil and Russia*. Oxford: Oxford University Press.
Almqvist, E., Adam, S., Bloch, M., Fuller, A., Welch, P., Eisenberg, D., Whelan, D., MacGregor, D., Meschino, W. and Hayden, M. (1997) Risk reversals in predictive

testing for Huntington's Disease, *American Journal of Human Genetics*, 61, 945–52.

Alper, J. (1996a) Biological influences on criminal behaviour: how good is the evidence? *British Medical Journal*, 310, 6975, 272–3.

Alper, J. (1996b) Genetic complexity in single gene diseases, *British Medical Journal*, 312, 196–7.

Alper, J. and Beckwith, J. (1993) Genetic fatalism and social policy: the implications of behavioural genetics research, *Yale Journal of Medicine*, 66, 511–24.

Anionowu, E.N. (1993) Sickle cell and thalassaemia: community experiences and oficial responses. In Ahmad, W.I.U. (ed) *'Race' and Health in Contemporary Britain*. Buckingham: Open University Press.

Asch, A. and Geller, G. (1996) Feminism, bioethics and genetics. In Wolf, S.M. (ed) *Feminism and Bioethics: Beyond Reproduction*. Oxford: Oxford University Press.

Beaudet, A. (1998) ASHG Presidential address. Making genomic medicine a reality, *American Journal of Human Genetics*, 64, 1–13.

Beck, U. (1992) *The Risk Society*. London: Sage.

Bekker, H., Modell, M., Nenniss, G., Silver, A., Mathew, C., Bobrow, M. and Marteau, T. (1993) Uptake of cystic fibrosis testing in primary care: supply push or demand pull? *British Medical Journal* 306, 1584–6.

Bell, J. (1998) The new genetics: the new genetics in clinical practice, *British Medical Journal*, 36, 618–20.

Billings, P., Beckwith, J. and Alper, J. (1992a) The genetic analysis of human behaviour: a new era, *Social Science and Medicine*, 35, 3, 227–38.

Billings, P., Kohn, M.A., de Cuevas, M., Beckwith, J. and Alper, J. (1992b) Discrimination as a consequence of genetic testing, *American Journal of Human Genetics*, 50, 476–82.

Board of Directors of the American Society of Human Genetics (1999) ASHG Statement Eugenics and the misuse of genetic information, *American Journal of Human Genetics*, 64, 335–8.

Bouchard, T. (1994) Genes, environment and personality, *Science*, 264, 1700–1.

Cantor, C. (1990) Orchestrating the Human Genome Project, *Science*, 248, 49–51.

Chapple, J. (1992) Genetic screening: brave new world or the boys from Brazil? *British Journal of Hospital Medicine*, 47, 7, 487–9.

Clarke, A. (1994a) The genetic testing of children. Report of a working party of the Clinical Genetics Society (UK), *Journal of Medical Genetics*, 31, 785–97.

Clarke, A. (1994b) Genetic screening: a response to Nuffield, *Bulletin of Medical Ethics*, 97, 13–21.

Clarke, A. (1995) Population screening for genetic susceptibility to disease, *British Medical Journal*, 311, 6996, 35–8.

Clayton, E., Hannig, V., Pfotenhauer, J., Parker, R., Campbell, P. and Phillips, J. (1996) Lack of interest by non pregnant couples in population-based cystic fibrosis carrier screening, *American Journal of Human Genetics*, 58, 617–27.

Conrad, P. and Weinberg, D. (1996) Has the gene for alcoholism been discovered three times since 1980? *Perspectives on Social Problems*, 8, 3–25.

Davison, C., Macintyre, S. and Davey Smith, G. (1994) The potential social impact of predictive testing for susceptibility to common chronic diseases—a review and research agenda, *Sociology of Health and Illness*, 16, 340–71.

Duster, T. (1990) *Backdoor to Eugenics*. London: Routledge.

Galton, D. and Galton, C. (1998) Francis Galton and eugenics today, *Journal of Medical Ethics*, 24, 99–105.

Giddens, A. (1991) *Modernity and Self-Identity. Self and Society in the Late Modern Age*. Cambridge: Polity Press.

Gieryn, T. (1983) Boundary-work and the demarcation of science from non-science: strains and interests in professional ideologies of scientists, *American Sociological Review*, 48, 781–95.

Gieryn, T. (1985) Boundaries of Science. In Jasanoff, S., Markle, G., Petersen, J. and Pinch, T. (eds) *Handbook of Science and Technology Studies*. Thousand Oaks, California: Sage.

Gieryn, T. (1999) *Cultural Boundaries of Science: Credibility on the Line*. Chicago: University of Chicago Press.

Gilbert, N. and Mulkay, M. (1984) *Opening Pandora's Box. A Sociological Analysis of Scientists' Discourse*. Cambridge: Cambridge University Press.

Gill, M. and Richards, T. (1998) Meeting the challenge of genetic advance, *British Medical Journal*, 316, 570.

Guston, D.H. (1999) Stabilizing the boundary between US politics and science: the role of the Office of Technology transfer as boundary organization, *Social Studies of Science*, 29, 1, 87–111.

Harper, P. (1992) Genetics and public health, *British Medical Journal*, 340, 721.

Harper, P. (1993) Clinical consequences of isolating the gene for Huntington's Disease, *British Medical Journal*, 307, 397–8.

Harper, P. and Clarke, A. (1995) Genetic testing for familial hypertrophic cardiomyopathy in newborn infants: testing may be unhelpful, *British Medical Journal*, 310, 6983, 856–9.

Harper, P. and Clarke, A. (1997) *Genetics, Society and Clinical Practice*. Oxford: BIOS.

Hartouni, V. (1991) Containing women: reproductive discourse in the 1980s. In Benley, C. and Ross, A. (eds) *TechnoCulture*. Minneapolis: University of Minnesota Press.

Heath, D. (1998) Locating genetic knowledge: picturing Marfan Syndrome and its traveling constituencies, *Science Technology and Human Values*, 23, 1, 45–70.

Hilgartner, S. (1990) The dominant view of popularization: conceptual problems, political uses, *Social Studies of Science*, 20, 519–39.

Hiller, E., Landenburger, G. and Natowitz, M. (1997) Public participation in medical policy making and the status of consumer autonomy: the example of newborn-screening programs in the United States, *American Journal of Public Health*, 87, 8, 1280–8.

Holtzman, N. (1997) Editorial: genetic screening and public health, *American Journal of Public Health*, 87, 8, 1275–7.

House of Commons Science and Technology Committee (1995) *Human Genetics: the Science and Its Consequence*. London: HMSO.

Hubbard, R. and Wald, E. (1993) Search for alcoholism gene ignores the complex genetics/environment interplay, *Genetic Engineering News*, July, 3–4.

Johnston, M. (1992) Precision of diagnosis in clinical genetics, *British Journal of Hospital Medicine*, 47, 7, 490–1

Juengst, E. (1996) Self-critical federal science? The ethics experiment within the U.S. Human Genome Project, *Social Philosophy and Policy*, 63–95.

Kamrat-Lang, D. (1995) Healing society: medical language in American eugenics, *Science in Context*, 8, 1, 175–96.

Keller, E. (1992) Nature, nurture, and the Human Genome Project. In Kelves, D., Hood, L. (eds) *The Code of Codes. Scientific and Social Issues in the Human Genome Project*. Cambridge, Massachusetts: Harvard University Press.

Kerr, A., Cunningham-Burley, S. and Amos, A. (1997) The new genetics: professionals' discursive boundaries, *Sociological Review*, 45, 2, 279–303.

Kerr, A., Cunningham-Burley, S. and Amos, A. (1998a) The new genetics and health: mobilising lay expertise, *Public Understanding of Science*, 7, 41–60.

Kerr, A., Cunningham-Burley, S. and Amos, A. (1998b) Eugenics and the new genetics in Britain: examining contemporary professionals' accounts, *Science, Technology and Human Values*, 23, 2, 175–98.

Kerr, A., Cunningham-Burley, S. and Amos, A. (1998c) Drawing the line: an analysis of lay people's discussions about the new genetics, *Public Understanding of Science*, 7, 113–33.

Kevles, D. (1986) *In the Name of Eugenics: Genetics and the Uses of Human Heredity*. Berkeley: University of California Press.

Khoury, M. and the Genetics Working Group (1996) From genes to public health: the applications of genetics technology in disease prevention, *American Journal of Public Health*, 86, 12, 1717–22.

Kinmouth, A., Reinhard, J., Bobrow, M. and Parker, S. (1998) The new genetics: implications for clinical services in Britain and the United States, *British Medical Journal*, 316, 767–70.

Lambert, H. and Rose, H. (1996) 'Disembodied knowledge'? Making sense of medical knowledge. In Irwin, A. and Wynne, B. (eds) *Misunderstanding Science? The Public Reconstruction of Science and Technology*. Cambridge: Cambridge University Press.

Ledley, F. (1994) Distinguishing genetics and eugenics on the basis of fairness, *Journal of Medical Ethics*, 20, 157–64.

Lippman, A. (1992a) Led (astray) by genetic maps: the cartography of the human genome and health care, *Social Science and Medicine*, 35, 1469–76.

Lippman, A. (1992b) Prenatal genetic testing and screening: constructing needs and reinforcing inequities, *American Journal of Law and Medicine*, 17, 15–50.

Lippman, A. (1993) Worrying—and worrying about—the geneticization of reproduction and health. In Basen, G., Aichler, M. and Lippman, A. (eds) *Misconceptions*, Vol. 1. Quebec: Voyageur Publishing.

Low, L., King, S. and Wilkie, T. (1998) Genetic discrimination in life insurance: empirical evidence from a cross sectional survey of genetic support groups in the United Kingdom, *British Medical Journal*, 317, 1632–5.

Ludmerer, K. (1989) American geneticists and the eugenics movement, 1905–1935, *Journal of the History of Heredity*, 30, 371–3.

McDermott, R. (1998) Ethics, epidemiology and the thrifty gene: biological determinism as a health hazard, *Social Science and Medicine*, 7, 9, 1189–95.

Macintyre, S. (1995) The public understanding of science or the scientific understanding of the public? A review of the social context of the 'new genetics', *Public Understanding of Science*, 4, 223–32.

MacKenzie, D. (1981) *Statistics in Britain, 1865–1930: the Social Construction of Scientific Knowledge*. Edinburgh: Edinburgh University Press.

Maddox, J. (1993) Has nature overwhelmed nurture? *Nature*, 366, 107.

Mahowald, M., Levinson, D., Cassell, A., Lemke, A., Ober, C., Bowman, J. *et al.* (1996) The new genetics and women, *The Milbank Quarterly*, 2, 143–57.

Marteau, T. and Richards, M. (eds) (1996) *The Troubled Helix: Social and Psychological Implications of the New Human Genetics.* Cambridge: Cambridge University Press.

Marteau, T., Johnston, M., Shaw, R.W. and Slack, J. (1989) Factors influencing the uptake of screening for neural tube defects and amniocentesis to test for Down's syndrome, *British Journal of Obstetrics and Gynaecology*, 96, 739–41.

Marteau, T., Drake, H. and Bobrow, M. (1994) Counselling following diagnosis of a foetal abnormality: the differing approaches of obstetricians, clinical geneticists and genetic nurses, *Journal of Medical Genetics*, 31, 864–7.

Mayeux, R. and Schupf, N. (1995) Apolipoprotein E and Alzheimer's Disease: the implications of progress in molecular medicine, *American Journal of Public Health*, 85, 9, 1280–4.

Michie, S., Bron, F., Bobrow, M. and Marteau, T. (1997) Non-directness in genetic counselling: an empirical study, *American Journal of Human Genetics*, 60, 40–7.

Nelkin, D. (1994) Promotional metaphors and their popular appeal, *Public Understanding of Science*, 3, 25–31.

Nelkin, D. and Lindee, S. (1995) *The DNA Mystique: the Gene as a Cultural Icon.* New York: W.H. Freeman and Co.

Nelkin, D. and Tancredi, L. (1989) *Dangerous Diagnostics: the Social Power of Biological Information.* New York: Basic Books.

Nuffield Council on Bioethics (1993) *Genetic Screening. Ethical Issues.* London: Nuffield Council on Bioethics.

Parsons, E. and Atkinson, P. (1992) Lay constructions of genetic risk, *Sociology of Health and Illness*, 14, 439–55.

Paul, D. (1992) Eugenic anxieties, social realities, and political choices, *Social Research*, 59, 3, 663–83.

Paul, D. (1995) *Controlling Human Heredity: 1865 to the Present.* New Jersey: Humanities Press.

Pembrey, M. (1998) In the light of preimplantation genetic diagnosis: some thical issues in medical genetics revisited, *European Journal of Human Genetics*, 6, 4, 4–11.

Pernick, M. (1997) Eugenics and public health in American history, *American Journal of Public Health*, 87, 11, 1767–72.

Petersen, A. (1998) The new genetics and the politics of public health, *Critical Public Health*, 8, 1, 59–71.

Plomin, R. and Craig, I. (1997) Human behavioural genetics of cognitive abilities and disabilities, *BioEssays*, 19, 12, 1117–27.

Plomin, R., Owen, M. and McGuffin, P. (1994) The genetic basis of complex human behaviours, *Science*, 264, 1733–9.

Press, N. and Browner, C.H. (1994) Collective silences, Collective fictions: how pre-natal diagnostic testing became part of routine prenatal care. In Rotherberg, K.H. and Thomson, E.J. (eds) *Women and Prenatal Testing: Facing Challenges of Genetic Technology.* Columbus: Ohio State University Press.

Quaid, K. and Morril, M. (1993) Reluctance to undergo predictive testing: the case of Huntington's Disease, *American Journal of Human Genetics*, 45, 41–5.

Rapp, R. (1998) Refusing prenatal diagnosis: the meanings of bioscience in a multi-cultural world, *Science Technology and Human Values*, 23, 1, 45–70.

Richards, M. (1993) The new genetics: some issues for social scientists, *Sociology of Health and Illness*, 15, 5, 567–86.

Richards, M. (1997) It runs in the family: lay knowledge about inheritance. In Clarke, A. and Parsons, E. (ed) *Culture, Kinship and Genes. Towards Cross Cultural Genetics.* Basingstoke: Macmillan Press.

Richards, M. and Ponder, M. (1996) Lay understanding of genetics: a test of a hypothesis, *Journal of Medical Genetics*, 33, 1032.

Rose, H. (1994) *Love, Power and Knowledge. Towards a Feminist Transformation of the Sciences.* Cambridge: Polity Press.

Rose, H. (1995) Social criticism and the Human Genome Programme: the limits of a limited social science, *The Genetic Engineer and Biotechnologist*, 15, 2–3, 164–79.

Rose, S. (1995) The rise of neurogenetic determinism, *Nature*, 373, 380–2.

Rothman, B.K. (1998) *Genetic Maps and Human Imaginations. The Limits of Science in Understanding Who We Are.* New York: W.W. Norton and Co.

Rues, V.I. and Freimer, N.B. (1997) Understanding of genetic basis of mood disorders: where do we stand? *American Journal of Human Genetics*, 60, 1283–8.

Savill, J. (1997a) Prospecting for gold in the human genome, *British Medical Journal*, 314, 43–5.

Savill, J. (1997b) Molecular approaches to understanding disease, *British Medical Journal*, 314, 126–9.

Schmidtke, J. (1994) Proceed with much more caution, *Human Genetics*, 94, 25–7.

Serra-Pratt, M., Gallo, P., Jovell, A., Aymerich, M. and Estrada, M. (1998) Trade-offs in prenatal detection of Down's Syndrome, *American Journal of Public Health*, 88, 4, 551–7.

Shakespeare, T. (1995) Back to the future? New genetics and disabled people, *Critical Social Policy*, 46, 22–35.

Sherman, S., De Fries, J., Gottesman, I., Loehlin, J., Meyer, J., Pelian, M., Rice, J. and Waldman, I. (1997) Behavioural genetics '97: ASHG statement. Recent developments in human behavioural genetics: past accomplishments and future direction, *American Journal of Human Genetics*, 60, 1265–75.

Smith, K. and Coyle, R. (1995) Attitudes towards genetic testing for colon cancer risk, *American Journal of Public Health*, 85, 19, 1435–8.

Sorenson, J.R. and Cheuvront, B. (1993) The Human Genome Project, health behavior and health education research, *Health Education Research*, 8, 589.

Stone, D. and Stewart, S. (1996) Screening and the new genetics: a public health perspectives on the ethical debate, *Journal of Public Health Medicine*, 18, 1, 3–5.

Sutton, A. (1995) The new genetic technology and the difference between getting rid of illness and altering people, *European Journal of the Genetics Society*, 1, 1, 12–20.

Sweeney, B. (1997) Genetic advances: great promise tempered with concern, *British Journal of General Practice*, 544–5.

Tsui, -C. (1992) The spectrum of cystic fibrosis mutations, *Trends in Genetics*, 11, 392–8.

Turney, J. (1993) Thinking about the Human Genome Project. Review article, *Science as Culture*, 282–94.

Wald, N., Kennard, A., Denrem, J.W., Cuckle, H.S., Chand, I. and Butler, I. (1992) Antenatal maternal screening for Down's Syndrome: results of a demonstration project, *British Medical Journal*, 305, 391–4.

Watson, J. (1990) The Human Genome Project: past, present and future, *Science*, 248, 44–9.

Wertz, D. and Reilly, P. (1992) Laboratory policies and practices for the genetic testing of children: a survey of the helix network, *American Journal of Human Genetics*, 61, 1153–68.

Wiesel, T. (1994) Editorial: genetics and behaviour, *Science*, 264, 1647.

Williamson, R., Allison, M., Bentley, T., Lim, S., Watson, E., Chapple, J. *et al.* (1989) Community attitudes to cystic fibrosis carrier testing in England: a pilot study, *Prenatal Diagnosis*, 9, 727–34.

Willis, E. (1998) Public health, private genes: the social context of genetic biotechnologies, *Critical Public Health*, 8, 2, 131–9.

Wilmut, I. (1998) Cloning for medicine, *Scientific American*, December, 30–5.

Working Party of the Clinical Genetics Society (UK) (1994) The genetic testing of children, *Journal of Medical Genetics*, 31, 785–97.

# 'Losing the plot'? Medical and activist discourses of contemporary genetics and disability

*Tom Shakespeare*

## Introduction

By a strange irony, the possibility of routine genetic intervention into human reproduction has coincided with the emergence of the disabled people's movement as a significant political player in many western societies. Just as the demand for civil rights and social inclusion has been placed on the political agenda, so the possibility has arisen of preventing the birth of foetuses affected with common genetic conditions. A major conflict has resulted, which is being played out via television documentaries, in magazines and newspapers, and occasionally through direct action by disabled activists. At the heart of this dilemma are the contested meanings of genetics and disability.

On the one hand, there is a narrative of genetic intervention as a major contribution to human health, and a new way of avoiding the suffering associated with impairment. On the other hand, there is a narrative of genetics as a totalitarian conspiracy to rid the world of disabled people.[1] This chapter explores these two major narratives, and contributes to the emerging literature on cultural discourses of genetics (Lippman 1994, Nelkin and Lindee 1995, Van Dijck 1998). There is a general absence of discussion of disability as the missing term in the debate around popular and scientific discourse of genetics (Shakespeare 1995). There are two particular gaps. The first is knowledge of the understandings that medical genetics practitioners have of disability and their attitudes towards disabled people. The second is disabled people's own views of genetic research and diagnostic screening.

While there have been some attempts to analyse and understand the relationship between the new genetics, particularly in terms of prenatal screening, and disability rights (Shakespeare 1995, Bailey 1996, Hubbard 1997, Shakespeare 1998b) these have centred on the extent to which the social practice of genetics could be said to be eugenic. As Paul (1992) has argued, the eugenics debate is irresolvable, because the label itself refers to a multiplicity of meanings. This chapter does not attempt to pronounce on the eugenic status of current genetics, but explores the ways in which opponents and proponents of genetics have represented new knowledge and new practices in their public rhetoric. The aim is to interrogate the particular narratives attached to genetic technologies by clinicians and disabled people, narratives in which the disavowal or accusation of eugenic intent plays a major role. In this sense, the chapter builds on the approach of Nelkin and Lindee:

> Commonly held beliefs about the power of the gene and the importance of heredity facilitate eugenic practices even in the absence of direct political control of reproduction, for eugenics is not simply gross coercion of individuals by the state; even in Nazi Germany, individual 'choice played a role in the maintenance of a highly oppressive state policy. Rather, it can be productively understood as a constellation of beliefs about the importance of genetics in shaping human health and behaviour, the nature of worthwhile life, the interests of society, and, especially, the meaning of reproductive responsibility (1995: 191).

Van Dijck suggests that we should view genetics as theatre or as performance (1998: 16), focusing her attention on aspects of staging such as characters, plots and performances. Thus she describes the common plot device of genetic discovery as a race (1998: 19) and the alternative invocation of fictional parallels, such as the Frankenstein or Brave New World stories (1998: 20). The title of this chapter draws on this critical cultural analysis approach, but also attempts to exploit the ambiguities in the term 'plot' itself. To suggest that medical clinicians and researchers have 'lost the plot' in terms of disability implies that they have failed to understand what disability is about, or what appropriate responses to the disability problem might be. Conversely, to suggest that some disabled activists should 'lose the plot' about genetics implies that there is a danger of equating all genetic research and practice with the historical precedent of Nazi eugenics, and of regarding geneticists as engaged in an authoritarian conspiracy to rid the world of disabled people.

Exploring the discourses of geneticists about disability, and of disabled people about genetics highlights what Van Dijck describes as 'the hybrid discourse of promise and concern' (1998: 51) which, she maintains, characterised early coverage of genetic research in the 1960s, and which is still prevalent today. There is a marked disparity between the generally upbeat, confident rhetoric of the genetics establishment and its media apologists, and the gloomy, hostile and suspicious reaction of disabled people and their organisations. Of course, it is not only disabled people who are concerned: environmentalists, religious figures, feminists and certain journalists share some of these anxieties. The point of the chapter is to examine critically geneticists' rhetoric about disability, and some disabled people's rhetoric about genetics. It is the author's argument that more dialogue between the two groups is urgently needed, and that clinical and technical information about genetic conditions needs to be complemented by social understandings of the experience of disability in contemporary society.

The chapter constructs two generalised categories, namely 'medical genetics' and the 'disability movement'. Clearly, these are imposed dichotomies and mask considerable variation of experience and attitude within each group. Within the medical group, for example, is included a range of medically-trained commentators, including genetic scientists, obstetricians, other clinicians and researchers, genetics counsellors, and even the occasional psychologist or bioethicist. 'Disability movement' refers to the network of self-organised disabled people's groups committed to the civil rights struggle. In Britain, this would mean organisations within the British Council of Disabled People, rather than the traditional charities or self-help groups (see Campbell and Oliver 1996, for a discussion of this political movement). Both doctors and disabled people are almost as unlikely to be in agreement with each other, as they are between themselves. It has been argued that geneticists, genetic counsellors and obstetricians hold differing positions on the issue of terminating pregnancy for foetal abnormality (Marteau *et al.* 1994), and disabled people range between those vigorously antipathetic to the new genetics (for instance those associated with BCODP), and those who welcome the promise of gene therapy to cure degenerative conditions (for instance, those associated with the Genetics Interest Group).

Furthermore, the chapter is itself a constructed narrative of the engagement of doctors and disabled people around genetics, from a particular standpoint. Just as many within the genetics establishment themselves occupy multiple roles as clinicians, researchers, advocates, writers, broadcasters and even sometimes business people, so disabled people may at the same time be people with a genetic condition, parents of people with a genetic condition, campaigners, advocates and researchers. Each individual, therefore, may simultaneously hold different perspectives or have different interests in the debate. There are multiple standpoints and competing accounts, but the purpose of this chapter is to try and untangle some of the ways in which rhetoric may operate to prevent communication and dialogue.

## Medical discourses around disability

Examples of gene rhetoric presented here are not the result of a systematic content analysis, but of a broad review of recent literature, including textbooks and major journals such as *American Journal of Human Genetics*, *Prenatal Diagnosis*, *Journal of Medical Screening*, *British Medical Journal* and other similar professional publications. It is clear from these public accounts, that clinicians and researchers are not espousing a clear-cut eugenic position, in most cases: as Kerr *et al.* found in their review of comparable literature.

The 'pro-genetics' argument tends to be carefully constructed and contains little or no evidence of blatant statements or views about the benefits of ridding society of genetically defective people (Kerr *et al.* 1998: 180).

This points to the limitations of relying on public pronouncements, and the need to try and gather more unguarded statements or undertake qualitative research. Methodologically, this raises a problem for disabled researchers, because it suggests that clinicians and researchers would present different accounts of their views to a disabled researcher than they might to someone seen as less implicated in the new technologies.

The way that ritual disclaimers operate has been highlighted by the medical geneticist Angus Clarke, in a reaction to a statement by his colleague Marcus Pembrey that reduction in the incidence of genetic conditions is not the object of genetic services:

> Sadly such statements from senior members of the profession are not enough: their wishing does not make it so. Those health professionals (often not clinical geneticists) who wish to adopt a public health perspective to justify our existence through a cost-benefit analysis will be quite capable of learning to preface their remarks by explicit, but purely cosmetic, disavowals of eugenic intent. It is often these cost-benefit considerations, with crude reckoning of cash saved per termination achieved, that speak loudest to health authorities (1991b: 1524).

Clarke goes on to castigate The Royal College of Physicians of London report on 'Prenatal Diagnosis and Genetic Screening' for just this combination of 'anti-eugenic' preface followed by a clear 'genetic hygiene' approach to inherited disease. Lippman has also referred to the genuflection towards the dangers of eugenics which is common in screening literature:

> Prenatal diagnosis necessarily involves systematic and systemic selection of fetuses, most frequently on genetic grounds. Though the word 'eugenics' is scrupulously avoided in most biomedical reports about prenatal diagnosis, except when it is strongly disclaimed as a motive for intervention, this is disingenous (1994: 147).

It would therefore be naïve to expect overt eugenicism in genetic discourse, with some exceptions (Wald *et al.* 1992, Shackley 1996, White 1997). Nevertheless, a clear set of values does emerge from the literature, which is implicit and subtle, but undoubtedly reflects a consensus that disability is a major problem, which should be prevented by almost any means necessary. Three dimensions of this proto-eugenic discourse will now be explored: narratives of tragedy; narratives of optimism; and ignorance about disabled people's lives.

*Narratives of tragedy*
First, it is possible to observe in discourses around genetic research and practice an implicit narrative or disability as personal medical tragedy. This is part of a broader discourse or disability in western culture (Oliver 1990,

Morris 1991), but is particularly strong in genetic discussions. For example, Abby Lippman talks about the way prenatal diagnosis is constructed as a way of avoiding 'disaster'. Genetics suggests that

> through the use of prenatal diagnosis women can avoid the family distress and suffering associated with the unpredictable birth of babies with genetic disorders or congenital malformations (1994: 146).

Again, Kerr and her colleagues found geneticists talking about the 'miserable lives' of disabled people (Kerr *et al.* 1998, 181).

In the papers examined, these attitudes are evident in the terms used. For example, the word 'risk' clearly has connotations of danger and negative outcomes. No one uses the word to describe the chance of winning the lottery. Other words include value-laden term such as 'burden', 'severe handicap', 'suffering', 'abnormality', and 'disorders', which are ubiquitous in this literature.

For example, Harper's classic textbook on genetic counselling talks about 'the burden of an affected child' (1981: 35). In an interesting, presumably subconscious, illustration of the equation that genetic abnormality equals disaster, Harper provides a Mendelian diagram of homozygosity in the autosomal dominant condition achondroplasia (restricted growth). The family tree has an affected mother and father with three offspring, two of whom are affected (heterozygotes), plus one sibling who is homozygous, and would die at birth. Yet clearly there is a fourth outcome: two affected parents have a 25 per cent risk of having a child who does not inherit the achondroplasia gene, and hence is of average height.

The idea that disabled people could be parents, or that a disabled baby might not inevitably be a tragedy is equally absent from the sweeping generalisation proposed by Jo Green and Helen Statham, who assert that:

> The discovery that a fetus has an abnormality may be seen either as a hazard or as a benefit of prenatal screening and diagnosis, but it is always devastating for parents (1996: 149).

In the same collection, another example of the tragedy discourse is provided by Marcus Pembrey's explanation of genetic science, which again uses phrases like 'disease gene', 'malfunction', 'causing all the trouble', 'mutant genes like this mess things up' (Pembrey 1996: 71). In a later article on pre-implantation diagnosis, he refers to selective termination as the lesser of three evils, the others being childlessness and the birth of an affected child (1998: 5) and to the 'terrible burden of having to choose' (1998: 7).

It is not suggested that these authors are extreme in their views, explicitly hostile to disabled people, or complacent about the past. For example, Harper (1992) warns about the history of eugenic abuse in the case of Huntington's Disease, and Pembrey (1998) is concerned that screening services should not have selective termination as the objective. These are liberal voices, anxious about abuse, yet equally certain that impairment is a terrible fate which should be avoided at all costs. But perhaps there is a continuum between the explicit eugenicism which Harper and Pembrey disown, and the mindset which views disabled people as a problem best prevented.

The particular words and phrases which are used in genetics debates reveal the implicit judgements which lie behind them. For example, Angus Clarke suggests, in relation to the Royal College of Physicians of London inquiry into genetic disorders, that

> Its very name clearly conveys the impression that the birth of any child with a genetic disorder represents a medical failure, at least until proved otherwise (1991a: 999).

Even those responsible for discovering the structure of DNA have reproduced this moral discourse, as when James Watson talks about 'bad genes' and 'culprit chromosomes' (1992: 167). Peter Conrad argues that this sort of 'gene talk' about 'bad' or 'defective' genes leads to the over-simplification of very complex issues, and problematic polarisation (1997). Deborah Lyn Steinberg discusses the construction of disease and disability through the lens of diagnostic genetics, in which:

> . . . genes seem to determine not only disease, but the negative social meaning of disease as an inevitable calamity. Moreover genetic disease is not only something terrible that someone has, but something someone is . . . In this context an 'offending gene' implicitly bespeaks an 'offensive' person, and is clearly implicated in the putatively imperative logic of genetic screening as a strategy to prevent the birth of persons with such 'diseases' (1997: 117).

*Narratives of optimism*
Clearly, if disability is regarded as being a terrible tragedy, the inevitable corollary is that the role of doctors is to cure it at all costs. From here it is a short step to suggesting that what cannot be cured (such as Down's syndrome), should be avoided in the first place. The discourse of genetics, therefore, centres on narratives of hope for affected families. In the popular press, but also in professional discourse, words like 'cure' and 'treatment' are used without any apparent irony, despite the fact that this 'cure' is actually to prevent the birth of the individual with the particular condition. For example, one of the criteria for introducing screening programmes is the availability of treatment (Health Departments of the United Kingdom, 1998). Yet the 'treatment' offered for conditions such as Downs syndrome is termination of the affected pregnancy. Equally John Bell writes:

> Genetic screening should be seen as a procedure used to alleviate human suffering resulting from all forms of human genetic disease (Bell 1990: 19).

Yet of course this alleviation of human suffering is achieved by eliminating the potential human.

A considerable literature documents how recent advances in genetic technologies such as the Human Genome Project, and particular methods of assisted conception and screening, have been greeted with hyperbole (Shakespeare 1995). This includes phrases like 'The Holy Grail' and 'The Book of Life'. Conrad talks about the ways in which media reports of genetic discoveries reflect a genetic optimism, comprising a belief that these will lead to treatments or the reduction of suffering (Conrad in press).

Wendy Farrant quotes the triumphalism of a *British Medical Journal* editorial on genetics, which proclaimed

> The antenatal diagnosis of fetal defects is perhaps the greatest advance in perinatal medicine for a generation (1985: 96).

This is part of the genetic discourse of optimism, which is upbeat about many issues without any apparent justification. For example, there is an optimism about the possibility of gene therapy despite 'only modest expectations of immediate clinical success' (Harris and Williamson 1996: 316, Dorin 1996).

There is optimism about the danger of genetic misuse: Wood-Harper and Harris speak enthusiastically about the potential of genetics, and complacently about the criticisms, dismissing feminist concerns with the phrase 'Such fears of eugenics becoming a social norm are probably unfounded' (1996: 282), after they have just outlined exactly that scenario. Pembrey (1998) is confident that increased selection of embryos will not lead to any backlash against disabled people, nor to more discrimination, nor to a reduction in facilities. He doesn't think there is any danger of the eugenic extension of selection termination or implantation.

There is also optimism about the practice of prenatal diagnosis, and considerable faith in the ability of affected women to make informed decisions after one-to-one counselling. Yet there is evidence that counselling may be unavailable or inadequate (Green 1994). For example, arrangements for informing women of screen negative results after tests for Down's syndrome have been shown to be inadequate: one research project found only 29 per cent of screening clinics had made specific arrangements, and in five per cent of cases these results were not given at all (Allanson *et al.* 1997). The Confidential Enquiry into Counselling for Genetic Disorders of the Royal College of Physicians found there was imperfect understanding and action on these issues (Harris and Williamson 1996). Belief in free choice and informed consent is therefore rather complacent (Shakespeare 1998b).

Above all, optimism is misplaced because, in the absence of any therapy, the only impact of genetic knowledge is to lead to selective termination or even sterilisation. For example, Harper argues:

Despite the recent arguments over the rights of the handicapped to reproduce, sterilization seems a perfectly reasonable course if the retardation is more than mild, the genetic risks high and the risk of pregnancy considerable (1981: 118).

Another commentator suggests:

. . . The long-term aim of genetic counselling is to see that as few people as possible are born with serious genetically-determined or part genetically determined handicaps (Carter 1979).

Again, screening trials show that, on average, 75 per cent of women accepted the offer of amniocentesis, and 92 per cent of women whose pregnancies were diagnosed as affected by Downs Syndrome chose to terminate (Haddow and Palomaki 1996).

Research suggests that obstetricians are significantly more likely to counsel termination of affected pregnancy than genetic specialists (Marteau *et al.* 1994). Research also implies that obstetricians are more directive in presenting prenatal screening tests (Marteau *et al.* 1993). As Farrant's research revealed, obstetricians often deploy eugenic arguments and believe it is their role to prevent impaired foetuses being born (Farrant 1985: 107). For example, one woman said:

The decision was made by the doctors. They said 'It's no use, the tests show it's abnormal. It's up to you what you do, but if you keep it you will live with the problem' (1987: 117).

It could therefore be suggested that protestations of clinicians regarding non-directiveness, consumer demand, and their neutrality on the question of disability should be heard with a great deal of scepticism. In particular, the narratives of cure and hope which abound in the literature, especially in the media reception of discoveries, conceal very limited options for those in receipt of the new genetic knowledge. Genetic discourses have a tendency to offer upbeat prognoses in a situation which involves considerable parental trauma (Green and Statham 1996, refer to the literature on psychological sequelae to abortion).

*Ignorance about disability*
There seems to be a significant imbalance in contemporary genetic discourses. That is, research creates ever more detailed knowledge of the human genome, of embryology, and of screening technology. Yet there is a deficiency in social and ethical understandings of the implications of technology and the appropriate responses to it. In terms of disability, there are two major areas of clinical ignorance which permeate the literature and contaminate the judgements made about desirable practices.

First, there is no clarity about what counts as disability, severe or otherwise. Clinicians resist attempts to construct a list of conditions for which screening might be allowed, arguing for consumer demand and the specificities of particular situations (Pembrey 1998). Yet this means that it is difficult at the same time for geneticists to suggest that there is a clear dividing line between appropriate and inappropriate criteria for screening and selective termination. At present, for instance, sex selection is regarded as inappropriate. Yet there is evidence that in other cultures (e.g. India), this is increasingly being seen as appropriate (Wertz and Fletcher 1998). The history of reproductive interventions suggests that the boundaries shift very quickly. Lee Silver (1998) hypothesises a future in which a wide number of social criteria are used as the basis for pre-implantation diagnosis, and in which access to technology is limited by ability to pay, and a genetic underclass results.

Clinicians reject this scenario out of hand, yet it is difficult to see wherein their confidence lies. At the current time, zygotes are being screened for late onset disorders such as colon cancer and Huntington's disease, and there is a debate about screening for breast and ovarian cancer (Wagner and Ahner 1998). Disabled commentators have demonstrated how disability is a social construction, a category with shifting boundaries (Shakespeare 1995), and this is an essential insight in the current era of expanding geneticisation. It might be inappropriate to stipulate the conditions for which screening is allowed, but it may be very appropriate to stipulate more explicitly the conditions for which screening is (or would be) prohibited. As Bernard Williams has argued:

> You cannot simply leave the question at the level of saying that modifying polygenetic traits by genetic means is technically highly improbable; you have to take it a stage further. The sensitive issue is how much further. It is a requirement on moral argument that it shouldn't simply stop at a mere technical fact, and say that the question doesn't arise . . . (Ciba Foundation 1990: 87).

There is a second area of medical ignorance about what it is like to be disabled. Sometimes, this is about simple clinical facts, such as how long people with cystic fibrosis are likely to live (Britton and Knox 1991). Many of those people who make pronouncements or policies based on how particular impairments are 'dreadful', are not the doctors who work closely with people and families affected. Moreover, it is very rare in the literature to hear the voice of people affected, which is a major absence in knowledge. Decisions are made as to the need for selective termination, yet there is ignorance about what it is like to live with a particular condition. This is a general problem of public, media and clinical discourse on genetics (Shakespeare 1998b):

> Clearly the investment of genetic disease with the spectre of an inevitably terrible life and early death fuels the sense that genetic screening is not

only necessary but the only possible response. In this context, the fact that actual experiences of these and other 'inherited illnesses' vary considerably is eclipsed, as is the possibility that the problems of 'disability' are not biologically determined but produced through oppressive social responses to illness and disability (Steinberg 1997: 118).

The point that clinical knowledge is not supplemented by sociological understanding or personal testimony can be expanded to highlight the ways in which disabled people have redefined disability. Approaches in disability studies focus on the social and structural production of disadvantage, rather than the individual consequences of impairments. The social model approach suggests that people are disabled by society, not by their bodies (Oliver 1990). The corollary is that the effective way to reduce disablement is to reform social organisation, not remove people with impairment from the population (Shakespeare 1995). As Lippman argues:

> Social conditions are as enabling or disabling as biological conditions. Why are biological variations that create differences between individuals seen as preventable or avoidable while social conditions that create similar distinctions are likely to be seen as intractable givens? (1994: 160).

## Disabled discourses about genetics

Given the ubiquity of contemporary genetic research and practice, and the way in which a narrative of disability as tragedy and screening as cure is presented, it is not surprising that disabled people have reacted with suspicion and anger. Excluded from debates, regarded as unfortunate misfits, it is entirely understandable that disabled people should be distressed and hostile (Stacey 1996: 344).

Yet, while it is vital to provide alternative perspectives, to challenge the prejudices and ignorances documented above, and to reveal the power imbalances inherent in society, it seems also incumbent on disabled radicals to provide an unemotional and balanced critique of the genetic project. It is important to undermine triumphalist genetic rhetoric by deploying evidence and reason, not by producing another equally ungrounded account.

Within much disability movement writing on genetics, it is possible to detect a common narrative theme. This is the reading of genetics as a preplanned plot against disabled people. For example, a bioethics supplement of the international newsletter *Disability Awareness in Action* talked about disabled people as:

> the target group for a 'search and destroy' mission, both before and after birth, incorporating highly effective technologies (DAA 1997: 1).

This highly emotive language is not entirely without foundation. However, in constructing a conspiracy story, it seems to overstate the case and reduce complexity to a dangerous uni-dimensionality. This 'plot' narrative rests on overuse of the Nazi metaphor, and a denial of the relevance of impairment.

*Equation of geneticists with Nazis*
No discussion of genetics can entirely avoid the historical experience of Nazi euthenasia and eugenics: this is a feature of a variety of social analyses, and is an important starting point for contemporary evaluations. For example, Ruth Hubbard argues:

> Our present situation connects with the Nazi past in that once again scientists and physicians are making the decisions about what lives to 'target' as not worth living by deciding which tests to develop. Yet if people are to have real choices, the decisions that determine the context within which we must choose must not be made in our absence—by professionals, research review panels, or funding organizations (1997: 200).

For example, many have raised the spectre of Nazi eugenics as a reminder of what can go wrong with attempts to improve the health of the population (Bailey 1996: 144). This seems legitimate. Several points should always be remembered: the fact that eugenic ideas were popular in pre-1939 Britain, America and other European countries as well as in Germany; the fact that German eugenics and euthenasia programmes were developed and implemented by leading doctors, rather than fascist stormtroopers; and the fact that some five per cent of the German population were sterilised, and approximately 275,000 murdered on the grounds of 'racial hygiene' (Burleigh 1994). Like the Holocaust or the Gulag, these historical events provide a testament to the lethal effects of a combination of authoritarianism and social prejudice: they cannot be brushed aside.

Yet, it is more dangerous to develop parallels between Nazi programmes and contemporary policies (DAA 199: 1), or directly to equate present genetic practice with previous authoritarianism. As historian Robert Burleigh suggests:

> Anyone who has discussed these issues will know that feeling of weariness when, inevitably, someone accuses their opponent of holding Nazi-like opinions on these issues, a charge which elicits an easy emotional response whether in the form of outrage or nods of eager approbation. In some circles, one needs simply to invoke Nazi Germany in order to touch base in terms of the unassailable authenticity of one's arguments (Burleigh 1997: 145).

Yet this practice is very frequent in the writings of disabled commentators:

Disabled people know only too well they are not welcomed in society, but the active promotion of abortion on the grounds of disability and determining that euthanasia is a viable proposition for the disabled foetus/child—is fascism (Rock 1996: 124).

Again, the activist Mike Higgins stated, in a speech at the opening of a City Council exhibition connected with disability and eugenics in Leeds, Yorkshire, that

The Nazis and their successors of today have made it acceptable to carry out the murder of disabled people and to discuss whether or not it should be extended.

By this he seemed to mean not just neo-fascist thugs, but also the genetics establishment.

Another example is the reaction of disabled people to the International Centre for Life, a combined genetics visitor centre and research centre in Newcastle, Tyne and Wear. Local activists of the disabled people's Direct Action Network carried out a demonstration at the building in 1997, using the slogan 'No Nazi Eugenics!', and Disability Action North East handed out a leaflet on 11 March 1998 which used phrases such as:'eugenic agenda', 'Nazi-style programme of the Geneticists', ' "virtual eugenics" theme park', and suggested that

Geneticists desperately want to exploit disabled people . . . so they can achieve even greater power within the ranks of the medical empire and over society at large.

While there are genuine and significant dangers of the extension of genetic research and practice, as outlined previously, it is unhelpful and insulting to see most clinicians as fascists or megalomaniacs. The extremism of such radical positions make it easier for geneticists and policy-makers to ignore the valid element of critique, and exclude disabled people from debates.

The final quotation above highlights another dimension of the 'plot' discourse, which is the way critics impart an intentionality and coherence to the genetic project which it does not necessarily possess. The conspiratorialism feeds the idea of a plan by the state, abetted by science, to eliminate all disabled people. Yet genetic advances are incremental, haphazard, contested and complex. Science is partial, unreliable, incomplete and sometimes inaccurate, despite the hyperbole of researchers.

Moreover, consumer demand plays a significant role in the adoption of genetic testing. The rhetoric of choice is central to the modern practice of genetics. The role of prospective parents has largely been ignored by disabled radicals. Because these are predominantly non-disabled people, it is likely that they will hold some of the prejudicial attitudes to disability which are common in society. Yet the decision to terminate pregnancy is not one that the majority of people take lightly. Moreover, there are reasons to want to prevent the birth of a child affected by impairment which do not reflect discrimination against disabled people: for example, the desire to avoid the early death or suffering of a loved child, or a feeling that a family will be unable to cope with the strain of looking after a very impaired member. Often it is prospective parents, not clinicians, who are the active partners in choosing to terminate pregnancy.

Therefore when disabled activists argue that:

> Disabled people are under threat for their existence in our modern technological societies. Medical science feels able to flex its muscles and power to abolish all life where the unborn foetus may be imperfect or impaired (Rock 1996: 121).

or that:

> Disabled people as a distinct group are specifically targeted before they are born. Access to prenatal diagnosis has for many years been driven by the goal of getting rid of certain groups of disabled people, for example those with Down's syndrome or spina bifida (DAA 1997: 1).

they are producing a narrative which locates control firmly with doctors, not pregnant women; which suggests that screening is motivated by a eugenic urge to eliminate disabled people; and which obscures the way in which it is women, and their partners, who are taking responsibility for difficult decisions about these pregnancies. Yet this is grossly to simplify the complexities of the ante-natal encounter. As has been argued elsewhere, eugenic outcomes may be an emergent property of the new genetics, but there is no evidence of an explicit plan to rid society of particular groups (Shakespeare 1998b).

Paul (1992) shows that the debate as to the eugenic nature of contemporary genetics is not ultimately resolvable, because the term 'eugenics' has so many meanings. Historically, the eugenic movement included those who favoured voluntary action, as well as those who called for state policy to prevent dysgenic reproduction. Yet it could be argued that many 'free' choices may be implicitly influenced or shaped by the medical personnel and the clinical context in which they are made. Also there is no clarity as to those practices which are not eugenic in intention, but may be eugenic in outcome. After all, the total effect of many individual decisions may be to remove disabled people from the population.

The complexities of these issues undermine the sloganising which equates genetics with eugenics, or doctors with Nazis. Complacency about the context in which reproductive decisions are made is misguided. Liberal scientists may facilitate the development of illiberal policies. Yet it is unhelpful and insulting both to physicians, and to those women and men who take the responsibility for making highly difficult choices for their families, to use highly emotive rhetoric to denounce modern ante-natal screening, and those who hold different moral positions on abortion or disability.

### Denial of impairment

It is clear that 'plot' narratives of genetics are ultimately an obstacle to a coherent critique of genetic research and policy, however appealing they may be to people with a sense of righteous indignation and anger. Yet there is another weakness of the disability critique which is perhaps more salient in the long term. This is the failure of the social model of disability to take account of the salience of impairment in the lives of many disabled people. There is a danger, in the stress laid on social and environmental barriers and practices, of ignoring the impact of physical and intellectual limitation and suffering on people lives (Shakespeare 1998a).

This weakness has been highlighted by a number of feminist disabled writers (Morris 1991), particularly Liz Crow. She argues:

> Instead of tackling the contradictions and complexities of our experiences head on, we have chosen in our campaigns to present impairment as irrelevant, neutral, and sometimes, positive, but never, ever as the quandry it really is (1996: 208).

This failure of disability radicals to engage with the lived experience of impairment tends to undermine the opposition posed to genetic practices which threaten to eliminate impairment. It could even be suggested that if disability is about social relations, not physical or intellectual impairments, then there can be no grounds logically for opposing the elimination of those impairments (Shakespeare 1998a).

Oliver rebuts these criticisms. He argues that the social model is about disability (social restriction), and that while he is not against talking about impairment, this must take place in a separate social model of impairment. He suggests that neither the social model of disability, nor his proposed social model of impairment, is a fully fledged social theory, and therefore it is invalid to criticise the social model of disability as being incomplete or unbalanced (Oliver 1996).

Of course, not all the disabled critiques of genetics are as crude as the ones highlighted. There are examples of sophisticated, nuanced and balanced analyses of the relationship between genetics and disability (e.g. Bailey 1996, Wolbring 1998). The draft position statement of the British Council of Disabled People, for instance, supports a woman's right to choose but opposes research which only seeks to increase pre-natal screening, not therapy. However, the 'genetics as Nazi plot' narrative is arguably the dominant voice in the disability movement at present.

Both the radicalism of the critique, and its simplistic emotionalism, provide parallels with the work of FINNRAGE (Feminist International

Network against New Reproductive Technologies and Genetic Engine-ering). As Hilary Rose observes, FINNRAGE became marginalised both because of its uncompromising oppositionalism, but also because its posi-tion was incompatible with the reality of women's lived experience (Rose 1995). This critique is echoed by Denny's research with women undergoing in vitro fertilisation, which leads her to challenge radical feminist accounts of the new technologies (Denny 1994). It suggests that there is a need to fos-ter broader research on the views of disabled people, including those with and without genetic impairments, and within and without the disability movement.

## Conclusion

As prenatal screening for more and more conditions is offered to more and more pregnant women, the cultural construction of genetics and disability develops an even greater significance. Because every pregnant woman will have to choose to what extent she avails herself of the diagnostic opportuni-ties which new technologies offer, the ways in which conception and preg-nancy, embodiment and impairment are presented become critical. A much wider debate is needed over issues such as the extent to which intervention may be desirable, and the quality of life available to people with particular impairments. This debate should not rely on the narrow expertise of geneti-cists, but should draw on the knowledge and experiences of different stake-holders.

Once the excitement has abated, perhaps both the opportunities and the threats from genetic intervention will be found to have been exaggerated. Yet there seems to be a curious parallelism between the discourses of medical genetics and disabled radicals. Both discourses seem to overstate the potential of genetics to impact on the lives of disabled people. The for-mer promises gloriously to eliminate impairment from the world, without seeming to understand or appreciate that this means eliminating people with impairment from society. The rhetoric of salvation through genetics regards prenatal conditions as illnesses like any other. Yet, as Bailey observes:

> This obscures the fundamental difference between prenatal testing and any other way of preventing illness, namely that the 'treatment' which follows prenatal testing—abortion—'cures' the condition by eliminating the foetus rather than by stopping the condition occurring in the first place [1996: 149].

The latter also seems to accept the geneticists' claim about their ability to remove impairment from the world. It suits a conspiracy theory approach to regard genetics as ubiquitous and all-powerful. But radicals react angrily to what they see as the plot to prevent disabled people from being born, without appreciating any benefits that there might be to reducing the incidence of certain impairments. On either side, hyperbole interrupts dialogue, and an appreciation of the ways in which technologies are being implemented, and decisions are being made.

It is important to point out that there are impairments and impairments. Tay-Sachs disease is more debilitating than Down's syndrome; cystic fibrosis is more limiting than achondroplasia. As Liz Crow argues:

> Impairment is problematic for people who experience pain, illness, shortened lifespan or other factors. As a result, they may seek treatment to minimise these consequences and, in extreme circumstances, may no longer wish to live (1996: 217).

This highlights the need for both disabled people and clinicians to understand the issue of impairment more effectively. This is not to say that people with a particular condition are less valuable than others, but to observe that some conditions limit life and cause significant suffering, while others do not. Particularly, degenerative conditions may impact more than static conditions, which may explain why some people with Friedrich's Ataxia have been amongst the keenest supporters of genetic research (Euro-Ataxia 1996). It is necessary to investigate these issues closely, rather than to assume that a particular condition is either unproblematic, or totally tragic.

Medical writers (Pembrey 1998) often argue strongly against any list of conditions for which selective termination or implantation may be permitted, while others attempt to distinguish between severe handicap, moderate handicap and mild handicap, and to offer termination only for moderate to severe handicap (Yagel and Anteby 1998). The UK Human Fertilisation and Embryology Authority already operate a list of suitable conditions for pre-implantation genetic diagnosis (Christine Godsden, personal communication). Disabled people will rightly want to contest both the construction and application of the particular categories, but may welcome a list of conditions for which screening is prohibited.

This type of debate highlights the need for information and dialogue between disabled people and medical professionals. There is a need for clinical information to be supplemented by information about disability, such as the literature now emerging in the disability studies field. Decisions about screening should be based on good information: rather than evaluating screening programmes in terms of those who undergo tests and terminations, programmes should be evaluated in terms of the proportion of people who were empowered to make an informed choice about their pregnancy (Marteau and Anionwu 1996: 124). This also implies the need for a disabled voice in debates, and to accept that disabled people, not doctors, are the real experts on disability, because of their personal experience of living with impairments.

In conclusion, this chapter has argued that it is possible to react with anger and opposition to the positions and practices of contemporary genetics, while not succumbing to the dangers of an equal and opposed rhetorical extremism. To resort to conspiracy theory is to undermine the ethical and sociological basis of critique. It also ignores the agency and responsibility of pregnant women and their partners. On the other hand, genetic hyperbole fails to respect the diversity of human embodiment, and the moral value of disabled people, as well as overstating the power of genetic intervention. Nuanced and balanced accounts of the potential and the dangers of contemporary genetic research and practice are urgently required.

A focus on narrative, begun in this chapter, shows the ways in which both geneticists and disabled radicals are constructing particular versions of genetics and disability. Attention to these accounts is important in the assessment and evaluation of particular proposals for policy and action. Lippman argues:

> Consequently, is is imperative that we continue to listen to the stories being told about prenatal testing and screening with a critical ear, situate them in time and place, question their assumptions, demystify their language and metaphors and determine whether, and to what extent, they can empower women (1994: 164).

I would suggest that it is both women and men, disabled people and non-disabled people, geneticists and non-geneticists, who should be listening and speaking carefully.

## Note

1   In Britain, the preferred term is 'disabled people', signifying that people with impairments are disabled by an exclusionary society: the American term 'people with disabilities' may put the individual first, but it still defines them by their impairment.

## References

Allanson, A., Michie, S. and Marteau, T.M. (1997) Presentation of screen negative results on serum screening for Down's syndrome: variations across Britain, *Journal of Medical Screening*, 4, 21–2.

Bailey, R. (1996) Prenatal testing and the prevention of impairment: a woman's right to choose? In Morris, J. (ed) *Encounters with Strangers: Feminism and Disability*. London: Women's Press.

Bell, J. (1990) Prenatal diagnosis: current status and future trends. In Ciba Foundation Symposium 149, *Human Genetic Information: Science, Law and Ethics*. Chichester: Wiley.

Britton, J. and Knox, A.J. (1991) Screening for cystic fibrosis (letter), *The Lancet*, 388, 1524.

Burleigh, M. (1994) *Death and Deliverance: 'Euthenasia' in Germany 1900–1945*. Cambridge: Cambridge University Press.

Burleigh, M. (1998) *Ethics and Extermination: Reflections on Nazi Genocide*. Cambridge: Cambridge University Press.

Campbell, J. and Oliver, M. (1996) *Disability Politics: Understanding our Part, Changing our Future*. London: Routledge.

Carter, C.O. (1979) Recent advances in genetic counselling, *Nursing Times*, 75, 1795–9.

Ciba Foundation Symposium 149 (1996) *Human Genetic Information: Science Law and Ethics*. Chichester: Wiley.

Clarke, A. (1991) Is non-directive genetic counselling possible? *The Lancet*, 388, 998–1001.

Clarke, A. (1991) Non-directive genetic counselling (letter), *The Lancet*, 388, 1524.

Conrad, P. (1997) Public eyes and private genes: historical frames, news constructions and social problems, *Social Problems*, 4, 2, 139–54.

Conrad, P. (in press) Media images, genetics and culture: potential impacts of reporting scientific findings on bioethics. In Hoffmaster, B. and A. Wylie (eds) *Bioethics in Context*. Cambridge: Cambridge University Press.

Crow, L. (1996) Including all of our lives: renewing the social model of disability. In Morris, J. (ed) *Encounters with Strangers: Feminism and Disability*. London: Women's Press.

Denny, E. (1994) Liberation or oppression? Radical feminism and in vitro fertilisation, *Sociology of Health and Illness*, 16, 1, 62–80.

Dorin, J. (1996) Somatic gene therapy, *British Medical Journal*, 312, 232–4.

Disability Awareness in Action, Special Supplement (1997) *Life, Death and Rights: Bioethics and Disabled People*. London: DAA.

Euro-ataxia (1996) Newsletter Number 11, European Federation of Hereditary Ataxias.

Farrant, W. (1985) Who's for amniocentesis? The politics of prenatal screening. In Homans, H. (ed) *The Sexual Politics of Reproduction*. London: Gower.

Green, J. (1994) Serum screening for Down's syndrome: experiences of obstetricians in England and Wales, *British Medical Journal*, 309, 769–72.

Green, J. and Statham, H. (1996) Psychosocial aspects of prenatal screening and diagnosis. In Marteau, T.M. and Richards, M. (eds) *The Troubled Helix*. Cambridge: Cambridge University Press.

Haddow, J.E. and Palomaki, G.E. (1996) Similarities in women's decision making, *Prenatal Diagnosis*, 16, 1161–2.

Harper, P.S. (1981) *Practical Genetic Counselling*. Bristol: John Wright and Sons.

Harper, P.S. (1992) Huntington Disease and the abuse of genetics, *American Journal of Human Genetics*, 50, 460–64.

Harris, R. and Williamson, P. (1996) Confidential enquiry into counselling for genetic disorders, *Journal of the Royal College of Physicians of London*, 30, 4, 316–17.

Health Departments of the United Kingdom (1998) *First Report of the National Screening Committee*, Department of Health.

Hubbard, R. (1997) Abortion and disability: who should and who should not inhabit the world? In Davis, L. (ed) *The Disability Studies Reader*. New York: Routledge.

Kerr, A., Cunningham-Burley, S. and Amos, A. (1998) Eugenics and the new genetics in Britain: examining contemporary professionals' accounts, *Science, Technology and Human Values*, 23, 2, 175–98.

Lippman, A. (1994) Prenatal genetic testing and screening: constructing needs and reinforcing inequities. In Clarke, A. (ed) *Genetic Counselling: Practice and Principles*. London: Routledge.

Marteau, T.M., Plenicar, M. and Kidd, J. (1993) Obstetricians presenting amniocentesis to pregnant women: practice observed, *Journal of Reproductive and Infant Psychology*, 11, 3–10.

Marteau, M., Drake, H. and Bobrow, M. (1994) Counselling following diagnosis of foetal abnormality: the differing approaches of obstetricians, clinical geneticists, and genetic nurses, *Journal of Medical Genetics*, 31, 863–7.

Marteau, T.M. and Anionwu, E. (1996) Evaluating carrier testing: objectives and outcomes. In Marteau, T.M. and Richards, M. (eds) *The Troubled Helix*. Cambridge: Cambridge University Press.

Morris, J. (1991) *Pride against Prejudice*. London: Women's Press.

Nelkin, D. and Lindee, M.S. (1995) *The DNA Mystique: the Gene as a Cultural Icon*. New York: W.H. Freeman.

Oliver, M. (1990) *The Politics of Disablement*. London: Macmillan.

Oliver, M. (1996) *Understanding Disability*. London: Macmillan.

Paul, D.B. (1992) Eugenic anxieties, social realities, and political choices, *Social Research*, 59, 3, 663–83.

Pembrey, M.E. (1996) The new genetics: a user's guide. In Marteau, T.M. and Richards, M. (eds) *The Troubled Helix*. Cambridge: Cambridge University Press.

Pembrey, M.E. (1998) In the light of preimplantation genetic diagnosis: some ethical issues in medical genetics revisited, *European Journal of Human Genetics*, 6, 4–11.

Rock. P.J. (1996) Eugenics and euthenasia: a cause for concern for disabled people, particularly disabled women, *Disability and Society*, 11, 1, 121–8.

Rose, H. (1995) Social criticism and the Human Genome Programme: some reflections on the limits of a limited social science, *The Genetic Engineer and Biotechnologist*, 15, 2–3, 169–79.

Shackley, P. (1996) Economic evaluation of prenatal diagnosis: a methodological review, *Prenatal Diagnosis*, 16, 389–95.

Shakespeare, T. (1995) Back to the future? New genetics and disabled people, *Critical Social Policy*, 44/5, 22–35.

Shakespeare, T. (1998a) Social constructionism as political strategy. In Velody, I. and Williams, R. (eds) *The Politics of Constructivism*. London: Sage.

Shakespeare, T. (1998b) Choices and rights? Eugenics, genetics and disability equality, *Disability and Society*, 13, 5, 665–81.

Silver, L. (1998) *Remaking Eden: Cloning and Beyond in a Brave New World*. London: Weidenfeld and Nicholson.

Stacey, M. (1996) The new genetics: a feminist view. In Marteau, T.M. and Richards, M. (eds) *The Troubled Helix*. Cambridge: Cambridge University Press.

Steinberg, D.L. (1997) *Bodies in Glass: Genetics, Eugenics, Embryo Ethics*. Manchester: Manchester University Press.

Van Dijck, J. (1998) *Imagination: Popular Images of Genetics*. Basingstoke: Macmillan.

Wagner, T.M.U. and Ahner, R. (1998) Just a choice or a step in the wrong direction, *Human Reproduction*, 13, 5, 1125–6.

190   Tom Shakespeare

Wald, N.J., Kennard, A., Denrem, J.W., Cuckle, H.S., Chand, I. and Butler, I. (1992) Antenatal maternal screening for Down's syndrome: results of a demonstration project, *British Medical Journal*, 305, 391–4.

Watson, J. (1992) A personal view of the project. In Kevles, D.J. and Hood, L. (eds) *The Code of Codes: Scientific and Social Issues in the Human Genome Project*. Cambridge: MA: Harvard University Press.

Wertz, D.C. and Fletcher, J.C. (1998) Ethical and social issues in prenatal sex selection: a survey of geneticists in 37 nations, *Social Science and Medicine*, 46, 2, 255–73.

White, C. (1997) Screening for fragile X is cost effective and accurate, *British Medical Journal*, 315, 205–10.

Wolbring, G. (1998) Submission to Health Canada: Renewal of Canadian Biotechnology Strategy, unpublished document of Council of Canadians with Disabilities.

Wood-Harper, J. and Harris, J. (1996) Ethics of human genome analysis: some virtues and vices. In Marteau, T.M. and Richards, M. (eds) *The Troubled Helix*. Cambridge: Cambridge University Press.

Yagel, S. and Anteby, E. (1998) A rational approach to prenatal screening and intervention, *Human Reproduction*, 13, 5, 1126–8.

# DNA identification and surveillance creep

*Dorothy Nelkin and Lori Andrews*

## Introduction

A wad of spit, a spot of blood, a semen stain, or a single hair is all that is necessary to create a DNA 'fingerprint'. DNA profiles can be extracted not only from blood or sperm at a crime scene, but also from objects touched by a person's hands, and from saliva used to lick stamps. From a tiny sample of body tissue, a forensic laboratory can create an image on an autoradiogram; a cluster of horizontal bands form a pattern, resembling a bar code. Despite its imperfect accuracy rate, law enforcement officials argue that DNA fingerprinting can be a unique way of identifying people and thus should be used as the gold standard.

DNA analysis had been developed in a medical context as a technique to identify the markers that indicate familial disorders. But in 1983, a British geneticist used the technique to identify a rapist. Subsequently, DNA testing spread out of the medical sphere into the sphere of public surveillance. As a non-intrusive and easy procedure, DNA fingerprinting has been used in many nonmedical contexts. It appeals to military, law enforcement and other governmental authorities: those seeking evidence to establish the identity of a dead body, a missing person, a biological relative, or the perpetrator of a crime. In 1990, the US Congress authorised and funded a military programme mandating the collection of blood and tissue for DNA testing of all military personnel. The FBI and the law enforcement agencies in every state require convicted felons to have a sample of their body tissue banked and tested for purposes of future identification. In some states, non-violent offenders and misdemeanants are included. Some countries require immigrants to provide a DNA sample as a condition of entry. DNA samples are collected and stored for the identification of missing children, or elderly Alzheimer's victims, or babies switched at birth, or genetic fathers in child support and paternity disputes. Men have brought their children to genetics clinics and had them secretly tested to determine if they were the 'real' fathers or if their wives had had an affair. The collection of body fluids for DNA identification is an expanding enterprise. At least 50 commercial DNA testing centres have been established in response to identity quests. A mail order company is selling a 'Defender DNA' device. If a perpetrator comes close, the potential victim jabs a pin into the attacker, activating an alarm and gathering an identifying DNA sample.

There are, of course, many reasonable purposes for DNA identification. Why not facilitate crime control by having records of recidivists? Why not develop accurate means of identifying missing persons or the remains of soldiers killed in war? To the military and law enforcement officials who collect body fluids for DNA identification, body material is an efficient means to implement legitimate policy goals. But the expanding use of DNA identification also reinforces a pervasive trend towards increased surveillance.

The early development of computer data systems attracted sociological attention to the possibilities and problems of growing surveillance. James Rule (1974) warned of institutional trends in which powerful bureaucracies would collect and store information on private persons to control their behaviour. He predicted a future of increasingly efficient mass surveillance and control. Michel Foucault conceptualised surveillance as a means of 'normalization' and focused attention on the production of knowledge in the service of power. Tests, he wrote, have become a means to 'compare, differentiate, hierarchize, homogenize, exclude' (1979: 183–4). Responding to the expansion of national information systems in the 1980s, Kenneth Laudon (1986) warned about the implications of a 'dossier society' for personal privacy and civil rights. Gary Marx focused on the use of these powerful data collection and data sharing tools in undercover police work, warning of 'almost imperceptible surveillance creep' marked by subtle, invisible, involuntary forms of social control (1988: 2). Criminologist David Garland (1995) takes a different view, arguing that surveillance technologies are essential and inevitable in complex societies that require formalised systems of data gathering. In his view, they are not in themselves the problem; rather, the issue is how they can be regulated to avoid abuse.

However, the development of DNA tests and banking systems has intensified concerns about surveillance technologies. For DNA samples, more than just a source of identification, can reveal information about a person's health and predispositions. How will organisations and political systems use DNA identification? Who will have access to the data? How can those in control of DNA data appropriately balance the identification benefits of this technology while protecting the social values of individual freedom and privacy? DNA databanking may be a useful tool for fighting crime and meeting military exigencies, but it is also subject to abuse for political or economic ends.

This chapter describes the gradual expansion of mandatory genetic testing for DNA identification. We focus on the disputes that develop when those required to provide DNA samples raise concerns about loss of benefits, psychological harm, and discrimination based on the information revealed by their DNA. And we use these disputes to analyse the problems of 'surveillance creep' as growing numbers of people have their DNA on file (McEwen and Reilly 1994).

## The military DNA collection programme

In January 1995, Corporal Joseph Vlacovsky and Lance Corporal John Mayfield III, two Marines stationed at the Kaneohe base near Honolulu, were ordered to provide blood and cheek epithelial cell samples as part of the military's mandatory genetic testing programme. Their DNA samples would be stored at the Department of Defense DNA Repository in order to facilitate the efficient identification of the remains of soldiers killed in battle. They refused to comply and were court-martialled for violating an order from their superior officer (Mayfield v. Dalton 1995). They became 'the first DNA conscientious objectors'.

The Department of Defense (DOD) began collecting blood and tissue from every person in the military services in 1992. Included in this programme are all active duty and reserve personnel as well as civilian employees and contractors, even though these persons are much less likely to become unknown soldiers. The tissue is collected, analysed, and then stored in the DOD's DNA Repository in Gaithersburg, Maryland. Each individual is provided with two sealed plastic cards that have a fingerprint, signature, blood stain and oral swab, and a bar code; the cost of this kit, pencil included, is $3.00 (not including the cost of analysing the DNA). DNA samples are vacuum sealed and frozen to ensure their survival for 40 years. When needed, bits of bodies can be identified by matching their DNA to the samples kept on file. By 2001, over 4 million tissue samples from military personnel will be in the Maryland repository. It is the largest DNA bank in the world.

Military authorities regard the identification of remains as a compelling interest for soldiers and their families. In every war, the military has established departments to identify the dead, and have developed techniques to assist in identification. Lt. Col. Victor Weedn, the initial programme manager of the Armed Forces DNA Identification Laboratory, is a forensic pathologist—a lawyer, MD, and expert on DNA analysis. He had used DNA techniques to identify the skeletal remains of Czar Nicholas II, the victims recovered from TWA Flight 800, and the members of the Branch Davidian cult killed in the fire in Waco, Texas.

Weedn explains the importance of a mandated military testing programme: 'It's an issue to the soldiers, sailors and airmen. They want to know that—if they pay the ultimate sacrifice—they will be remembered' (Weedn 1996). He talks about the effectiveness of DNA identification and the time it would save in the slow and painful task of identifying human remains. He hopes to make the Tomb of the Unknown Soldier a thing of the past.

The problem of identifying remains was a major issue during World War I, with its devastating death toll and enormous number of bodies that had been dismembered beyond identification (Bourke 1996). The dead body of the 'unknown soldier' became a potent symbol of the horror of war. But Vlacovsky and Mayfield cared less about the identification of their dead bodies than their ability to control the integrity of their living bodies. Explaining his willingness to risk a court-martial, Vlacovsky said: 'This won't destroy the rest of my life. When this is over, I will still have control over my DNA'.

The Marines argued in court that the taking of their tissue violated their Fourth Amendment right to privacy. They regarded the requirement as unreasonable search and seizure: 'I expected to give up some privacy when I joined the military', said Mayfield. 'But,' he added, 'It doesn't say we hereby waive our constitutional rights'. 'It is our God-given right to maintain possession of our genes' (Mayfield 1995). Having little trust in military authorities, they also suspected that the tissue samples would be misused or used without their knowledge or consent for purposes other than the identification of their remains. Samples could be used to assess soldiers' predisposition to homosexuality (Hamer and Copeland 1994), or to a genetic disease and then used against their personal interests. Or their DNA could be used for purposes they oppose, such as the development of biological weapons (Cole 1996). And the information collected from their DNA samples could be available to law enforcement authorities in criminal investigations.

The Council for Responsible Genetics and a clinician, Paul Billings, submitted affidavits supporting the objecting Marines. They documented cases where access to genetic information revealing predisposition to genetic disease had resulted in discrimination. 'Thousands of tests could be done on these samples', Billings said: 'The military may have kept the door open as a way to counteract rising benefits costs by excluding coverage for those with pre-existing conditions that can be discovered in DNA samples' (Billings 1995).

Weedn dismissed such concerns: 'When you've licked a stamp on your tax return you've sent the government a DNA sample' (indeed, FBI had tested the saliva on postage stamps to link a suspect to the World Trade Center bombing and to identify the Unabomber). Weedn insisted that 'each specimen is treated as a medical specimen with confidentiality and respect'. Questioned about the initial DOD policy of keeping specimens after service members were discharged from the military—a policy later changed—he replied that it would be 'extremely costly and time consuming to return or destroy the specimens' (Weedn 1996). Instead, Weedn called for greater trust; he said he would not abuse the information in the DNA files.

Weedn's plea for trust did not convince the Marines. 'With nuclear testing, they just handed people some dark glasses and said "here, watch the bomb go off" . . . In the 1950s they gave LSD to army troops . . . In the 1970s they sprayed Agent Orange over their troops' (Chadwin 1996). Trust could hardly have been strengthened when Assistant US Attorney Theodore Meeker dismissed the importance of informed consent: 'If the military's use of unproved drugs on its personnel does not require informed consent, collection and storage of blood samples and oral swabs for possible use in identifying human remains does not require consent' (Meeker 1995).

Though both Vlacovsky and Mayfield had exemplary service records, they were threatened with court-martial proceedings, incarceration, fines, and dishonourable discharge for refusing to obey orders., However, a military judge dropped the charges in light of the fact that there were no existing regulations dealing with the consequences of failing to comply with the programme. Thus, both Marines received honourable discharges with veterans benefits—and they kept their DNA.

By the time of the decision, however, they had become interested in the general issues raised by mandatory testing. So Vlacovsky and Mayfield filed a civil suit in the District Court in Hawaii against the DOD on behalf of all service personnel claiming that the military programme ignored existing protocols for confidentiality and consent. The court dismissed their suit, contrasting the 'hypothetical' arguments of the Marines to the 'compelling interest' of the military to account for its troops. The court held that the taking of a blood sample was not unreasonable seizure and thus did not violate the Fourth Amendment. Taking blood was, after all, legally considered a minimal intrusion. And, because there was no immediate plan to use the specimens for research, the Nuremberg Code's requirements for informed consent were not relevant.

The DOD did amend the rules for its original banking programme. They reiterated that the samples would only be used for the identification of human remains unless they were subpoenaed for a criminal investigation or 'other uses compelled by other applicable law'. The programme was accelerated—testing of all current military personnel, including civilian employees, was to be completed by 1999.

Other cases quickly followed. In April 1996, Sgt. Warren Sinclair, age 33, a 14-year Air Force veteran and medical equipment repairman, refused to submit blood samples for genetic testing. Vlacovsky and Mayfield generally mistrusted military motives, but Sinclair, an African American, had specific political concerns about the use of his body tissue. He was convinced that DNA samples would be used to support racist claims. 'Would we ask Jews to give their genes to Germans? No. . . . Until the issue of racism is resolved, Afro-Americans should maintain possession of their genetic material' (Sinclair 1996). Sinclair recalled the use of genetic testing in the 1970s when blacks in the Navy were tested for sickle cell carrier status. Though no scientific evidence suggests this would affect a person's health (only reproductive decisions), those found to be carriers were disqualified from certain jobs. Black servicemen interpreted the exclusion as one more way to restrict their opportunities.

The Air Force court ruled against Sinclair, arguing that the interest of the government in assuring the identification of remains outweighed the intrusiveness of taking blood. Sinclair was convicted by court-martial on 10 May 1996 and sentenced to 14 days of hard labour and a two-grade reduction in rank (US v. Sinclair 1996).

In April 1996, Donald P. Power, a 1st Class Petty Officer and Navy nuclear technician, refused to give a DNA specimen because it violated his religious principles as a member of a Native American Lodge. Power said: 'My body is a sacred recipe to me, and I didn't think I should share it . . . They were not holding a part of me on a shelf. . . . You find personal power in knowing who you are' (Hinde 1997). For his refusal, Power lost a stripe, his security classification, and 40 per cent of his income. He applied for a waiver on grounds of religious freedom and it was accepted 18 months later. But few members of the armed services will be able to make use of the narrow religious exception, and moral objections are not enough to avoid military rules.

Those who refused to comply with mandatory genetic testing were challenging longstanding assumptions about the authority of the military over the bodies of its men. The military, after all, sends bodies into battle and soldiers cannot refuse assignments that threaten their bodily integrity. Refusal was in effect a declaration of rights based on a view that DNA holds special meaning for the individual; it was beyond the usual domain of military intrusion. As one of the Marines put it: 'It's your genetic blueprint, how you were created. . . . Your body is one of the few things that you have control over'. Moreover, the Marines mistrusted the promises of confidentiality; they believed that their samples would become a useful and efficient resource not just for identification purposes, but for decisions about promotion, health insurance, and law enforcement.

## DNA dragnets

Since World War II, law enforcement agencies have been expanding their information systems. But until the 1960s, many record-keeping systems functioned on the basis of local tradition, and the management of criminal justice information was uneven. By the late 1960s, the increasing sophistication of computers converged with growing fear of crime to encourage experiments with identification and surveillance systems (Marx 1988). In 1968, President Johnson's Commission on Law Enforcement and the Administration of Justice declared that information and systems technology was the most important tool for controlling crime. The Commission also proposed the creation of a national computerised criminal history repository.

But the efforts to implement a system faced public opposition. Attitude surveys suggested that Americans had little confidence in institutional leaders, mistrusted centralised information systems, and feared the implications for liberty and privacy (McClosky and Brill 1986). The idea of a national identity centre raised fears that growing government surveillance would extend well beyond the criminal justice system. Critics emerged to warn of the potential for abuse, the unwarranted tracking of 'suspicious' persons, the selective surveillance of particular groups, the harassment of political activists, and the leakage of information to private organisations seeking information for employment or credit ratings.

Although proposals to collect and bank human tissue for DNA identification raise similar issues, there has been remarkably little protest against them. Indeed, they have been welcomed as an effective means to lower the cost of criminal investigations. People may worry that computer banks store information on their economic status or credit rating, but few believe that the collection of DNA samples will affect their personal interests. And the aura of science underlying DNA technologies contributes to the legitimacy of testing and overrides privacy concerns.

However, those who are directly affected by mandatory genetic testing have responded by using the courts to challenge the programmes. In 1991, six inmates from Virginia's Tazewell Correctional Unit Number 31 challenged the state's mandatory DNA testing programme (Jones v. Murray). Virginia, in 1989, had been the first state to require the collection of blood samples from convicted sex offenders and felons for use in a state DNA database. Law enforcement officials attempted to justify the programme by citing a study indicating high recidivism rates.

The inmates claimed that the Virginia programme was unconstitutional; that in the absence of individualised suspicion, mandatory extraction of DNA samples violated their Fourth Amendment right against search and seizure. Also, they argued, imposing blood test requirements as a condition of release would impose additional punishment for their crimes and interfere with the right to due process by putting extra conditions on possibilities of parole.

Like soldiers, prisoners relinquish certain rights. But the prisoners defined their right to bodily integrity in a distinctive category; their body fluids, their genetic blueprint, should not be violated even in the context of the prison system. The Virginia Court disagreed. It conceded that the state could not meet the standards of probable cause or individual suspicion. But the court balanced the government interests in deterring and detecting crime against the privacy interests of inmates, and found the law to be reasonable. Convicted felons, said the court, already lose the right to privacy from routine searches of the cavities of their bodies and their prison cells. Most searches, however, are conducted to determine whether the inmates present a current danger—by, for example, concealing weapons. In contrast, the collection of DNA is to protect against a remote future risk.

Dissenting, Circuit Judge Murnaghan concurred with the decision as applied to violent felons, but lambasted the idea of collecting blood from prisoners who had been convicted of nonviolent crimes and who thus were unlikely to commit violent crimes in the future. He questioned whether the lack of reasonable expectation of privacy in a prison cell should extend to permit searches of the body fluids of every felon, violent and nonviolent alike. Perhaps most important, Judge Murnaghan suggested that 'The only state interest offered by the Commonwealth for including non-violent felons is administrative ease'. Reviving the 1980s concerns about the social implications of creating computerised criminal history systems, Murnaghan expressed 'a deep, disturbing and overriding concern that . . . the Commonwealth may be successful in taking significant strides towards the establishment of a future police state, in which broad and vague concerns for administrative efficiency will serve to support substantial intrusions into the privacy of citizens' (Murnaghan 1992).

Other states also began to develop DNA identification programmes, and in 1993, the FBI implemented CODIS, a national programme to assist federal, state, and local law enforcement agencies, support development of a population statistical data base, improve DNA forensic analysis methods, and serve humanitarian purposes such as the identification of missing persons or the human remains from mass disasters. The FBI promoted CODIS on the grounds of 'productivity and efficiency'. Former Director of the FBI crime laboratory, John Hicks, had described the computer databank as 'nothing more than an information management and screening tool' (Hoeffel 1990). He expected that 'It will save time and effort, and courts will have fewer cases to process because investigations can be better focused and coordinated' (FBI 1991). CODIS links the DNA profiles of convicts gathered by scattered law enforcement DNA labs, encourages uniform standards, and pools DNA data to facilitate identification of criminals across borders. The 1994 Crime Control Act reinforced these efforts through a provision for coordinating nationwide DNA databank systems. A report, commissioned by the Justice Department to implement the Act, announced an award of $8.75 million in grants to states and city crime agencies to improve their DNA testing capabilities (Butterfield 1996). As a result of that incentive, all 50 states have adopted laws requiring specified offenders to provide blood samples for forensic DNA testing.

State statutes vary. Most statutes initially required that saliva and blood samples be obtained from sex offenders on their release from prison, or as a condition of probation or parole. Statistically, sex offenders do have a high rate of recidivism. Strategically, selecting a group with such a negative public image for mandatory DNA testing was unlikely to provoke objections. Once in place, the DNA programmes expanded to cover a range of both violent and nonviolent crimes. In New York, blood samples are taken from defendants convicted of felony, sex offence, felony assaults, incest, or prison escape. In Virginia, those convicted of mail fraud must also store samples, and Mississippi law includes persons convicted of elder abuse. In Wisconsin, if a judge determines that a crime 'might have escalated to a sex crime' he can require registration. At least seven states test misdemeanants.

Provisions for access to criminal data banks also vary; the most restrictive statutes allow access only for law enforcement purposes. Maintaining confidentiality is also problematic: there are over 19,000 law enforcement agencies in the US and over 51,000 additional criminal justice agencies worldwide, which means over 600,000 employees have direct access to the National Crime Information Center maintained by the FBI.

Law enforcement agencies also enjoy access to many other DNA sources. The military had admitted it is willing to release its data to law enforcement officials (Gill 1997: 185). A proposed federal law, the Human Genome Privacy Act, would allow police officers to have access to hospital diagnostic DNA collections without patient authorization (Pear 1996). It is easier for police investigators to gain access to medical records than to bank records, e-mail information, or video-rental receipts—all of which are protected by federal privacy statutes.

Yet law enforcement purposes can be very broadly defined. Indeed, what is a law enforcement purpose? Would it include the identification of a man who failed to provide child support? Ohio explicitly allows its databank to be used pursuant to a court order for proceedings establishing paternity or maternity. Laws in New Jersey and Maryland allow their DNA banks to be used to find genetic parents where the party seeking to search the databank has obtained a court order.

DNA data could also be used to explore whether an individual has a genetic profile that might predispose him to aggressive acts (Andrews 1998). Both political parties have made crime a priority issue and state legislatures are granting money to build more and higher security prisons in the hopes that this will reduce crime. There is increased discussion in the popular and policy media about predicting and preventing crime by identifying those people thought to have 'criminal genes' (Nelkin and Lindee 1995). Information that purports to identify those 'predisposed' to violent behaviour holds considerable policy appeal. Yet many innocent people could be snared in the law enforcement net if their genes suggested they were potentially violent.

The military and prisons are self contained, or what sociologist Erving Goffman called 'total institutions' that operate under special rules with respect to social control and the right to intrude on the privacy of individuals (Goffman 1961). But the attraction of efficiency has also encouraged a wider use of DNA fingerprinting as DNA dragnets are used to search for suspects in serious crimes. These may involve many innocent people.

In 1990, the San Diego police department collected blood samples from 800 men during a search for a serial killer. They selected men who matched the description of a 'dark-skinned male'. In 1993, the two-year-old daughter of an American Army Sergeant stationed in Germany was kidnapped, raped, and murdered. The murderer was identified after an eight-month dragnet investigation that included DNA screening of 1900 men who had been near the military housing complex (Atkinson 1995). In 1995, police in Prince George County, Florida, searching for a serial rapist, collected saliva samples from more than 2300 men, stopping them at random on a road near the scene of the crime. In 1998, 50 hospital employees were asked to provide saliva samples in a dragnet search for the strangler of a popular nursing administrator. The police chief, John S. Farrell explained his use of the DNA dragnet:

'It is a way to focus the investigation efficiently . . . in a more business like fashion. . . . It would save time and money [each DNA test cost only $30] . . . It is an extremely cost-effective tool' (Pan 1998). But the African Americans on the hospital staff felt they were targets of discriminatory suspicion.

In his dissent in Jones v. Murray (1992), Judge Murnaghan contended that efficiency is not a legitimate interest and could be used to justify the testing of any citizen on grounds that it might reduce administrative workloads. He worried that arguments for administrative efficiency could justify DNA testing of all citizens at birth simple because of the likelihood of some future manifestation of violence; even when there is no specific evidence this will occur. Murnaghan also pointed out that, if the state was willing to allow the collection of blood from nonviolent offenders, the same logic would allow 'the testing of other discrete populations, e.g. racial minorities or residents of underprivileged areas'. Under the majority's logic, the state could go into the inner city and demand blood samples.

A similar argument was effective in a Massachusetts case in which a court halted collection of DNA from inmates, probationers, and parolees on grounds that it violated Fourth Amendment Rights. Benjamin Keehn, a Boston Public Defender, had pointed to the slippery slope: 'Why not round up poor people? Poor people are more likely to have their DNA on file. Of course there are benefits every time you get a cold hit. There are going to be dramatic success stories. But where does it stop? Why not take DNA samples at birth?' (Keehn 1998).

Refusal to comply with requests to submit a blood sample in a DNA dragnet is bound to imply guilt. Submission to testing is not necessarily voluntary. In addition, the collection of body tissue for DNA testing presents a distinctive set of problems, for unlike fingerprints, tissue samples expose individuals to the risk that the cells will be used for purposes other than identification. They can reveal information about predisposition to disease or physical traits, a fact that becomes increasingly problematic as public authorities responsible for social control in an expanding range of situations—such as immigration—are attracted to DNA testing as a means to extend surveillance and facilitate investigations.

**Surveillance creep**

In 1989, the Thatcher government in Great Britain instituted a policy allowing officials to use DNA fingerprint tests on immigrant applicants seeking to prove they have relatives in Britain. Over the subsequent few years, 18,000 tests were carried out on immigrants. Most testing is done in UK consulates in the country of origin. DNA testing is considered a cheap and more effective alternative to hours of questioning. But the British testing programme was criticised as racially discriminatory, and as creating 'a bureaucratic barrier and financial barrier' to immigration. Officially, applicants have a right to refuse to be tested, but rarely do so. Many do not understand why British officials want their blood, and, as in DNA dragnets, the implications of refusal lead most people to comply (Evans 1995).

The practice of testing immigrants spread to Canada in 1991. The purpose of the Canadian policy was to help immigrants with inadequate documents reunite with their families. But the cost, borne by the families sponsoring immigrants, is high: the government charged $975 for the applicant and $325 for each relative sponsored. A national committee on the status of women called the immigrant testing programme a way to discourage Third World immigration. High priced tests resulted in differential application of immigration policies, thereby 'adding fuel to a growing tide of racism and anti-immigrant sentiment . . . It would be more fair for Canada to come out publicly and say we don't want family sponsorship any more rather than put up all kinds of ridiculous obstacles which cost so much money' (Rinehart 1995).

The United States has never required DNA testing for immigrants, but in the anti-immigration fervour of the 1990s, pilot projects were set in motion to develop worker ID cards that would be linked to an electronic data base. They would include fingerprints, voice prints, and DNA sequences—to assure that only citizens and legal aliens hold jobs (Davis 1995). Under the US Immigration and nationality Act of 1952, aliens can be excluded from immigration for mental or physical defects, diseases, or disabilities. Information about diseases, disabilities, and predispositions could be gleaned from the applicant's DNA and therefore used as a basis to deny the application. Should genetic testing, then, be required of all immigration applicants?

In an odd extension of genetic testing, an Israeli researcher applied DNA techniques to the identification of the true Cohanim—the Orthodox Jews who trace their lineage 3300 years back to the first high priest. He found a genetic pattern on the Y chromosome that is shared by the descendants of the Cohanim (Grady 1997). These descendants are accorded higher status and are the only rabbis to perform certain religious duties. A DNA test could be used to validate a presumption of priesthood.

As DNA replaces other technologies such as HLA blood typing or fingerprints, the collection and banking of body tissue for DNA analysis is becoming mandatory in more and more contexts. It is the preferred technology for identifying recidivists and remains, but its use is expanding.

Increasingly, it is not doctors or public health officials who collect tissue samples for identification, but government, law enforcement agencies, the military, and immigration authorities. Private firms are increasingly involved as collecting tissue becomes a growing business. One company, Identigene, advertises in taxis, subway cars, and bill boards (Call 1-800 DNA TYPE). It collects tissue for DNA identification (at $600) that can establish paternity in child support disputes or family relationships for immigration purposes. A phone call to the company suggests they have not considered questions about the privacy of stored samples or who should have access to them.

Greater efficiency and reduced costs are also encouraging the 'surveillance creep' that Marx (1988) had predicted. In 1998, a senior member of the British police force called for a national DNA testing data base of the entire population, arguing that it would cut the time and cost of investigating crimes (Gammon 1998). Techniques of DNA are improving and costs are declining. The Department of Justice expects that the average cost of a DNA test can be reduced to less than $10. Technological developments have also increased the feasibility of manufacturing DNA testing dogtags. A one-centimetre-sized chip can contain all the genetic information needed to identify 10s of thousands of genes at a time and to store them on a DNA card.

## Why worry?

At first glance, DNA identification programmes seem an efficient way of solving crimes, preventing immigration fraud, and identifying soldiers who die serving their country. The increased collection of DNA data and the expansion of centralised DNA banks have evoked little public response. It may seem comforting to law-abiding citizens who view the technology as resolving social problems with little relevance to themselves. But the cases described above suggest reasons for concern. Just as the targets of DNA fingerprinting have expanded, so too have the uses of DNA information. Yet, there are possibilities for error in the collecting and banking of DNA samples and many potentials for abuse. Innocent people can be snared in the DNA identification net.

### Possibilities of error

DNA fingerprinting has been called the 'gold standard' of identification. The technology is premised on the assumption that DNA fingerprints are unique for each individual. Indeed, a printout of a person's entire genome of more than three billion base pairs would be a unique identifier, except for identical twins. However, forensic tests look at only a small subset of a person's genome, and segments may be shared by other individuals especially within an ethnic group. Statistically, the chances that DNA from a crime scene actually comes from a particular suspect depends on how many other individuals could share that DNA pattern. Laboratories use a reference population of samples to assess the probability of a random match. However, selecting reference populations that are appropriately representative is often difficult (Lander 1994).

In addition, there is potential for laboratory error. Proficiency tests, used to check laboratory capabilities, have revealed many problems. In one proficiency test, a Cellmark analyst, instead of loading the two samples in different lanes, loaded the same sample in both lanes—and unwittingly declared a match where there was none. In a 1993 study, 45 laboratories were asked whether particular DNA samples matched. The labs were undoubtedly using their best techniques since they knew they were being tested. Yet, in the 223 tests performed, the study identified matches in 18 cases where matches did not exist (Koehler et al. 1995). If these had been real trials, innocent people would have been convicted.

In an actual case, the bloodstain found on the watch of a defendant seemed to match the blood from the victim, both showing three DNA bands. But the DNA from the watch showed two extra bands, not mentioned in the laboratory report. Rather than concluding that the accused individual might be innocent, the company decided that the sample probably included non-human contaminants. But, in an unusual move, genetic experts for both the prosecution and defence analysed the forensic DNA work and issued a joint statement that it was unreliable: 'If these data were submitted to a peer-reviewed journal in support of a conclusion, they would not be accepted', said the experts (Lander 1994: 197).

The interpretation of DNA fingerprints is also prone to bias. In a sociological study of forensic scientists, William Thompson documented ways in which the institutional context in which these scientists work influences 'the development and validation of new testing procedures, the interpretation of results, and their presentation in court' (Thompson 1997, 1117). Forensic scientists have professional incentives to adopt the goals of their clients and this may compromise scientific detachment. Keen on justifying the value of their services, they may be reluctant to question the reliability of tests. And in ambiguous situations, they may make interpretive errors (Thompson 1997).

In a study of responses to DNA evidence, University of Texas researchers set up a team of mock jurors (actually university students) and found they did not appreciate the importance of laboratory error rates. Jurors are often faced with 'misleading assurances from forensic science experts that laboratory errors are impossible or nearly impossible'. The study indicated to the researchers that DNA evidence 'could lead to conviction where acquittals might otherwise result' (Koehler et al. 1995).

Errors can also be a problem in the military context. To justify the use of DNA identification in the military, Lt. Col. Weedn argued that 15 to 30 per cent of previously collected fingerprint cards could not be used for identification because the cards were smudged. But DNA samples are no less prone to error and sloppy handling.

Changing methods of analysis open new possibilities of error, but neither the laws regulating forensic programmes nor those allowing court admission of DNA evidence provide adequate protection. 'Providing blanket admissibility for any type of DNA analysis whatsoever (as these loosely drawn statutes might appear to do) is an invitation for mischief', says geneticist Eric Lander (Lander 1994).

*Potentials for abuse*

In the cases we have described, plaintiffs feared their samples would be used for other than identification purposes, that military or forensic investigators might also look at health status and other information that could lead to genetic discrimination. To date, forensic DNA bankers have been able to claim they are testing only for identification purposes and that their samples could not be used for revealing health problems. But there are possibilities for abuse in the future: certain markers that were not thought to indicate medical risks may turn out to reveal health information. Some state forensic departments are buying used gene sequencers from companies, putting within their control the ability to sequence genes including those that indicate health risks.

Abuses are likely to increase as interest turns to behavioural genetics, for predictive information about behaviour may be useful in both military and criminal contexts. The uses of such data are likely to reflect existing stereotypes. The scenarios Judge Murnaghan presented are realistic. If genes associated with aggressive or criminal behaviour were identified, it would be easy to envisage selective testing of black men in light of current stereotypes associating crime with race. Numerous incidents of selective investigation suggest the way stereotypes might influence data banking practices. In Pennsylvania, state police instructed bank employees to photograph suspicious looking blacks, in effect, creating a criminal profile applying to specific race groups. Airport security profiles have also used race as an indicator of potential terrorism or drug smuggling crimes.

If genetic predispositions were identified for antisocial acts, social interests could encourage measures to prevent crime by circumscribing the rights of people thought to have criminal genes. This might include identifying those with antisocial genes, keeping them under surveillance, or preventively detaining them. Their profiles might be kept on file to be consulted when a crime is committed. In the military context, identification of genetic predisposition to homosexuality could—as the Marines suspected—have devastating consequences. Though the military may not directly ask, the genes may tell. Soldiers with that genetic makeup could simply be discharged even when there was no evidence they engaged in homosexual behaviour.

Concerns about such misuse of surveillance technologies are not without basis. In the 1960s and 1970s the FBI and local law enforcement officials kept tabs on thousands of citizens who were active in the civil rights and anti-war movements, and in some cases harassed innocent people. Today, the tools of surveillance are improving with the growing capacity of central data banks that include DNA. The Fourth Amendment might protect against secondary use of samples that were collected for purposes of identification, but this is a matter of dispute. Indeed, the concerns about privacy that had been raised by critics in the early days of centralised computer data banks are increasingly urgent when the data are DNA.

*Violations of privacy*

To the marines, prisoners, and immigrants who challenged mandatory testing, body tissue holds religious, social and political meanings, and privacy concerns were critical. For Native American Donald Power, the military's taking of DNA violated his religious beliefs. Mayfield and Vlacovsky defined their DNA in terms of personal identity. And even prisoners, whose privacy rights are compromised, defined the taking of DNA as different from the searching of prison cells or body cavities.

While convicted felons would have lesser rights than other individuals, the potential uses of forensic DNA banks affect more than just criminals. Those tested in a DNA dragnet because they happen to be in an area will then have their DNA samples on file. Victims also have their DNA tested at forensic labs and their samples may be banked. Family members related to the offenders are also affected because health information about the offender (say, a genetic predisposition to cancer) indicates genetic risks to relatives as well.

Collecting tissue samples from an individual who has not been charged or convicted of a crime—as in a DNA dragnet—could violate the person's Fourth Amendment right to be free from unreasonable searches and seizures. However, persuaded by the 'scientific' nature of 'profiling', courts have allowed the random stopping of individuals thought to fit criminal profiles of hijackers or drug smugglers. One judge, referring to a hijacker profiles as 'elegant and objective' was convinced that hijackers had characteristics 'markedly distinguishing them from the general traveling public' (US v. Lopez 1971).

As a controlling tool for modern institutions and complex organisations, the use of DNA is appealing. But in light of problems of privacy and potentials for abuse, testing should be closely regulated. The Fourth Amendment could be used to prohibit non-consensual tissue collection so as to limit the taking of DNA samples (Krent 1992). Informed consent doctrines could be more widely enforced to limit possibilities of abuse. Or the property interests in the body could be recognised, giving people greater control over what is done with their tissue (Andrews 1986). There could be greater limits on access to DNA information: Vermont legislation, for example, includes language in a databanking bill to prohibit the use of genetic information as a basis for employment and insurance decisions.

Though the practice of testing and banking DNA is extending to a widening range of people—from soldiers who go to battle to chaplain's assistants, from violent to nonviolent felons, from immigrant families to foreign adoptees—there has been little public concern about the practice. The possibilities of error are deflected by faith in science and, especially, the promise of genetics. Potential abuses of DNA data are deflected by perceptions that surveillance pertains to 'others'—the soldier, the criminal or the illegal immigrant—and a belief that DNA identification is an efficient means to maintain social order.

Moreover, Americans these days have few expectations of privacy, accepting surveillance in many spheres. Shoppers accept television surveillance in department stores, strollers accept camera surveillance in public parks (Nelkin 1995). The dossier society that Laudon and Rule predicted years ago has crept up on us; facilitated by the ability to gather, store, and access information—not just about finances, credit rating, or consumer preferences, but about the body, identity, and health.

In 1972, a legal scholar wrote that the social security numbers assigned to us at birth have become a 'leash around our necks, subjecting us to constant monitoring and making credible the fear of the fabled womb-to-tomb dossier' (Miller 1972). Could DNA identifiers eventually replace social security numbers, requiring every person to have DNA on file? Today, according to Janet Hoeffel (1990), 'It is not merely paranoia to imagine the incremental steps the current government would take that would lead from a data bank with DNA profiles on criminals to a data bank with profiles on each of us'. Indeed, molecular biologist Leroy Hood has predicted that within 20 years all Americans will carry a credit card type plastic stripe that contains computer readouts of their personal genomes: 'Your entire genome and medical history will be on a credit card' (Hood 1996).

## Acknowledgements

We wish to acknowledge the support of the National Science Foundation EVS Program grant #SBR-9710345, the assistance of Michelle Hibbert, and the comments of David Garland and David H. Kaye.

## References

Andrews, L. (1986) My body, my property, *Hastings Center Report*, October, 28–38.

Andrews, L. (1998) Predicting and punishing anti-social acts: how the criminal justice system might use behavioral genetics. In Rothstein, M. and Carson, R. (eds) *Behavioral Genetics and Society: the Clash of Culture and Biology*. Baltimore, MD: John Hopkins Press.

Atkinson, R. (1995) DNA samples catch American killer of toddler in Germany, *The Washington Post*, 1 January, A27.

Billings, P. (1995) Amicus in Mayfield v. Dalton 95- 00344.

Bourke, J. (1996) *Dismembering the Male: Men's Bodies, Britain and the Great War*. Chicago: University of Chicago Press.

Butterfield, F. (1996) US has plans to broaden availability of DNA testing, *New York Times*, 14 July.

Chadwin, D. (1996) The DNA war, *The Village Voice*, May, 14.

Cole, L. (1996) The specter of biological weapons, *Scientific American*, December, 62.

Davis, A. (1995) Digital IDs for workers in the cards, *National Law Journal*, 10 April, 17.

Evans, K. (1995) Targets of the genetic inquisition, *The Guardian*, 29 March, 12.

Federal Bureau of Investigation (1991) Legislative guidelines for DNA databases, US Department of Justice, November.

Foucault, M. (1979) *Discipline and Punish*. New York: Vintage Books.

Gammon, P. (1998) cited in UK police chief calls for national DNA data base, *Nature*, 393, 14 May, 106.

Garland, D. (1995) Surveillance and society, *CJM*, 20, Summer, 3–4.

Gill, S. (1997) The military's DNA registry: an analysis of current law and a proposal for safeguards, *Naval Law Review*, 44, 175–222.

Goffman, E. (1961) *Asylums*. New York: Anchor Books.

Grady, D. (1997) Who is Aaron's heir? *New York Times*, 19 January, 4.

Hamer, D. and Copeland, P. (1994) *The Science of Desire*. New York: Simon and Schuster.

Hinde, J. (1997) Their hands on your genes, *Times Higher*, 7 March, 19.

Hoeffel, J. (1990) The dark side of DNA profiling, *Stanford Law Review*, 42 January, 465–538.

Hood L. (1996) quoted in Garrett, Laurie The dots are almost connected, *Los Angeles Times Magazine*, 3 March, 49.

Keehn, B. (1998) quoted in Goldberg, Carey DNA databanks giving police a powerful weapon, and critics, *New York Times*, 19 February, A1, A12.

Koehler, J., Chia, A. and Lindsey, S. (1995) The random match probability in DNA evidence: irrelevant and prejudicial? *Jurimetrics*, 35, 201–9.

Krent, H.E. (1992) Of diaries and DNA banks: use regulations under the Fourth Amendment, *Texas Law Review*, 74, 49–100.

Lander, E. (1994) DNA fingerprinting, science law and the ultimate identifier. In Kevles, D. and Hood, L. (eds) *The Code of Codes*. Cambridge: Harvard University Press.

Laudon, K. (1986) *The Dossier Society*. New York: Columbia University Press.

Marx, G.T. (1988) *Undercover: Police Surveillance in America*. Berkeley: University of California Press.

Mayfield, J. (1995) quoted in Essoyan, S. Two marines challenge Pentagon order, *Los Angeles Times*, 27 December, A1.

McCloskey, H. and Brill, A. (1986) *Dimensions of Tolerance*. New York: Russell Sage Foundation.

McKewen, J.E. and Reilly, P. (1994) A review of state legislation on DNA forensic data banking, *American Journal of Human Genetics*, 54, 941–58.

Meeker, T. (1995) quoted in Essoyan, S. Two marines challenge Pentagon order, *Los Angeles Times*, 27 December, 5.

Muller, A. (1972) *The Assault on Privacy*. New York: New American Library.

Murnaghan, J. (1992). In *Jones v. Murray*, 962 F.2d. 302, at 313 (dissenting).

Nelkin, D. (1995) Forums of intrusion: comparing resistance to information technology and biotechnology. In Bauer, M. (ed) *Resistance to New Technology*. Cambridge: Cambridge University Press.

Nelkin, D. and Lindee, M.S. (1995) *The DNA Mystique: the Gene as a Cultural Icon*. New York: W.H. Freemen.

Pan, P. (1998) Prince George's chief has used serial testing before, *Washington Post*, 31 January, B01.

Pear, R. (1996) Clinton would broaden access of police to medical records, *New York Times*, 10 December.

Rinehart, D. (1995) DNA tests help not hinder relatives. *Montreal Gazette*, 10 May, A16.

Rule, J. (1974) *Private Lives and Police Surveillance*. New York: Schocken Books.

Sinclair, W. (1996) Memorandum to convening authorities, 27 June.

Thompson, W.C. (1997) A sociological perspective on the science of forensic DNA testing, *University of California Davis Law Review*, 30, 4, 1113–36.

Weedn, V. (1996) Stored biological specimens for military identification, Oberman Seminars, 14 June.

## Cases

*Jones v. Murray* (1992) 962 F 2d 402 (4th Cir.), cert. denied. 506 US 977.

*Mayfield v. Dalton*, 901 Fu. Supp. 300 (d. Hawaii 1991), vacated and remanded, 109 F. 3d 1423 (9th Cir 1997).

*US v Lopez* (1971) 328 F Supp. 1077, 1081.

*US v. Sinclair* (1996) (Central Judicial Circuit, USAF Trial Judiciary, 10 May).

# Notes on Contributors

Peter Conrad is Harry Coplan Professor of Social Sciences and Chair of the Department of Sociology at Brandeis University. He received his Ph.D. from Boston University and has published six books, including the award-winning *Deviance and Medicalization: From Badness to Sickness* (with Joseph W. Schneider), and dozens of journal articles and chapters. He is currently writing a book on how genetics and behavior has been reported in the news media over the last thirty years.

Susan Cox is a Post Doctoral Fellow in the Centre for Applied Ethics at the University of British Columbia. Her primary interest is interpersonal communication about hereditary illness. She is currently working on several related projects which focus on everyday morality and the experiences of families at risk from Huntington Disease, Autosomal Dominant Polycystic Kidney Disease, and Breast/Ovarian Cancer.

Sarah Cunningham-Burley is senior lecturer in medical sociology, Department of Community Health Sciences, University of Edinburgh. She has recently completed a study, along with colleagues Anne Kerr and Amanda Amos, on 'The Social and Cultural Impact of the New Genetics' funded under the ESRC Risk and Human Behaviour Programme. She is currently examining professional discourses on the social aspects of the new genetics, as well as work on disability and the new genetics.

Elizabeth Ettore is Reader in Sociology of Health and Illness at the University of Plymouth, England. After receiving her PhD from the London School of Economics, she worked at the Universities of London, Åbo Academy and Helsinki. She has directed research projects in the area of new genetics, ethics and prenatal screening. Her recent publications include: Women and Substance Use (1992); Gendered Moods (with Elianne Riska) (1995); and Women and Alcohol: from a private pleasure to a public problem (1997). She is currently working on a book, Reproductive genetics gender and the body, for Routledge.

Jonathan Gabe is a Senior Research Fellow in the Department of Social and Political Science at Royal Holloway, University of London. He has published in the areas of mental health, health care professions, health policy and the mass media and health. Currently he is involved in research on 'Violence against Professionals in the Community'. He is co-editor in Sociology of Health and Illness and editor of the journal's monograph series.

Nina Hallowell is a Senior Research Associate in the Centre for Family Research at the University of Cambridge. Her research interests include the psychosocial implications of new genetics technologies particularly the lay understanding of genetic risk and the implications of risk management.

Lesley Henderson is Research Fellow at the Mass Media Unit, Department of Sociology University of Glasgow. She has published on the production, content and audience reception of mass media coverage of health and social problems. She is currently researching the influence of media images of infant-feeding on women and will be undertaking a study of the role of media advocacy in tackling health inequalities.

Anne Kerr is currently doing research into the social history of cystic fibrosis (funded by the Wellcome Trust) and writing a book with Tom Shakespeare on genetics and eugenics. After her PhD studies on gender, feminism and science she worked on an ESRC project with Sarah Cunningham-Burley and Amanda Amos, with whom she has published a range of articles on professional, lay and media accounts of the new genetics.

Jenny Kitzinger was, until recently, based at the Glasgow University Media Research Unit. However, she has now taken up the post of Reader in Sociology at the University of Brunel, where she is developing a new centre for media and communications research. Jenny specialises in examining the media coverage and public understandings of social issues such as health, sexual violence and science. She is co-author of 'The Mass Media and Power in Modern Britain' (Oxford University Press); 'Great Expectations' (BfM press) and 'The Circuit of Mass Communication' (Sage). She is also co-editor, with Rose Barbour, of 'Developing Focus Group Research: politics, theory and practice' (1999, Sage).

Paul Martin is Research Fellow at the Genetics and Society Unit, School of Sociology, University of Nottingham. His recent research includes a study of the clinical and commercial development of gene therapy in Europe and the US, and work on the development of mammalian cloning. He is currently writing a book about the historical sociology of gene therapy technology.

William McKellin (Ph.D.) is a medical and linguistic anthropologist in the Department of Anthropology and Sociology, University of British Columbia. He has conducted research on the impact on families of genetic testing for Huntington disease, Alzheimer disease and hereditary cancer. Other research includes the impact of disability on families, and narrative and discourse analysis. He also teaches in the Faculty of Medicine at UBC and is a member of the Hereditary Cancer Program of the British Columbia Cancer Agency.

Dorothy Nelkin holds a University Professorship at New York University teaching in the Department of Sociology and School of Law. She is a member of the National Academy of Sciences Institute of Medicine, and author of Selling Science and (with Susan Lindee) The DNA Mystique. She is currently writing a book with Lori Andrews on disputes over body tissue in the biotechnology age.

Tom Shakespeare is a Research Fellow in the Disability Research Unit, University of Leeds. He is co-author of The Sexual Politics of Disability (Cassell, 1996), and Exploring Disability (Polity, 1999), and he edited The Disability Reader (Cassell, 1998). He has written and broadcast widely on issues of disability and genetics. He has a G to A transposition at point 380 of his FGFR3 gene.

Alan Stockdale is a medical anthropologist and a Senior Research and Development Associate in the Center of Applied Ethics and Professional Practice, part of Education Development Center, Inc., Newton, Massachusetts. Before joining Education Development Center he was a Fellow in the Program in Genomics, Ethics, and Society at the Stanford University Center for Biomedical Ethics.

# Index

ADY- 6408                                    4/13/01

ARMSTRONG

RB
155
S633
1999